Advance pr...
Staff Productiv...

"Jerry deserves to ... practice management that is chock-full of his vast experience and insight, yet simple, practical, and full of useful real-life examples. It's a step-by-step guide that any ambitious OD can easily follow and implement and, in doing so, ensure they'll meet the goals they set—all that, and a fun read as well!"

— ALAN GLAZIER, OD, FAAO - Founder, ODs on Facebook

"Jerry Hayes has done a great job of utilizing practical, real-world experiences based on triumphs and mistakes to guide practitioners from all practice sizes through his proven methods for success. His refreshing approach of straight talk and frank dialogue, along with his well-written and easy to read style, make this a must-have book for all optometrists. Most of all, I admire Jerry's unselfish passion to help others. He is unique, and so is this book. Get it! Read it!"

— HOWARD PURCELL, OD, FAAO - Senior VP of Customer Development for Essilor

"Dr. Jerry Hayes, my friend and business partner, is a brilliant entrepreneur with a proven track record of building successful companies. In this book, Jerry uses his down-to-earth writing style to share his vast knowledge and experience in staff management and team motivation. A must read for every optometrist in private practice, this book will help you make more money."

— NEIL GAILMARD, OD, MBA ,FAAO - President, Prima Eye Group, CEO Gailmard Eye Center

"This book combines a lifetime of business experience with meaningful data. Dr. Hayes shares his business experience and insights in a manner that is readily understood, and implemented. This is a practical message of 'how to' that provides a successful way to move to the next level of optometric practice!"

— BILLY COCHRAN, OD - Former President, Southern College of Optometry

"*How to Measure and Improve Staff Productivity in Private Practice* Optometry should be entitled, 'How to Break the Glass Ceilings of Private Practice Optometry.' Dr. Hayes, in a clear and concise manner, exposes the roadblocks to success that all Optometrists face in private practice. Each chapter is presented as a 'glass ceiling'—then, in a clear step-by-step manner, Dr. Hayes gives the reader the 'hammer' to break out of mediocrity. This is truly a must read for both new and seasoned practice owners!"

—HOWARD R. DAY, OD – Day Eye Care
Gardendale, AL

How to Measure and Improve Staff Productivity

in Private Practice Optometry

How to Measure
and
Improve Staff Productivity
in Private Practice Optometry

Jerry Hayes, O.D.

Copyright © 2014 by Jerry Hayes, O.D.

How to Measure and Improve Staff Productivity in Private Practice Optometry
First Edition, Paperback – published 2014

ISBN - 978-1500824884

ISBN - 1500824887

All rights reserved. No part of this book may be reproduced or transmitted in any form or by any means, electronic or mechanical, including photocopying, recording, or by any information storage and retrieval system without the written permission of the author, except where permitted by law.

Printed in the United States of America

Dedication

If I have seen further, it is only by standing on the shoulders of giants.

This book is dedicated to two men who were thought leaders and giants in optometry—the late Dr. Robert Koetting of St. Louis, MO, and Dr. Irving Bennett of Beaver Falls, PA. I am forever grateful for the examples they set, and the guidance they gave me when I was a young OD struggling to build a practice in small town Mississippi.

Acknowledgements

I was recently asked, "How do you do so much and still find time to write a book?" The honest answer is it's all about the team. I work hard to surround myself with results-oriented people who give me the support I so greatly need to get things done.

The person who deserves most of the credit for any success I have had is my wife and life partner of more than forty years, Cris Hayes. She keeps me healthy, happy, and organized. I love her dearly, and I appreciate her more than she will ever know.

Next, I want to thank the people who had a formative influence on my business thinking starting with consultant Carl Hicks, PhD of Jackson, MS. He was the person who first helped me realize that I could hire the talents and knowledge I didn't possess myself which was a life changing epiphany for me. Other consultants who played an important role in my development as a team leader were Pat

MacMillan and Jim Webb of Triaxia Partners in Atlanta, GA.

I am a former client and a huge fan of Dan Sullivan, CEO of The Strategic Coach program based in Chicago, IL. Dan claims to have coached more entrepreneurs than anybody in the world, and I have certainly benefited from his provocative way of looking at business, success, and life in general.

Lastly, I owe a big thanks to three colleagues at Prima Eye Group: my partner, Dr. Neil Gailmard, who is the President of Prima, Terri Abraham, who has a strong background in Human Resources and is an important part of the Prima success story, and my son, Nathan Hayes, who is Prima's Practice Finance Consultant. They all contributed greatly to the ideas presented in this book.

I would not be the person I am today without the influence all of these people have had on me.

Contents

Introduction 13

Chapter 1 23
   What Are Your Obstacles to Growth? 23

Chapter 2 35
   Doctor Productivity 35

Chapter 3 43
   How Big Does My Team Need to Be? 43

Chapter 4 57
   When Do You Need an Office Manager? 57

Chapter 5 67
   How Much Should I Pay My Staff? 67

Chapter 6 77
   Keeping Your Salaries in Line 77

Chapter 7 95
   Do Staff Bonuses Really Work? 95

Chapter 8 113
   Give Your Team a Sense of Purpose 113

Chapter 9 123
   Team Meetings 123

Chapter 10 134

Holding Your Employees Accountable 134
Chapter 11 153
   Hiring Top Performers 153
Epilogue 167
   Success Secrets of High Producing ODs 167

Introduction

Even though I've been writing and speaking on staff productivity since the early 1980s, over thirty years, it's fair for any reader to ask what qualifies Jerry Hayes to write a book on team productivity for optometrists?

My career as a staff manager started the same way it does for most private practice optometrists, as a one doctor, one assistant office. I made a lot of basic mistakes when a nice young lady named Betty was my one and only employee. One blunder that comes to mind is the lack of any written office policy. That created some hard feelings when Betty wanted to take off on a bank holiday that I had planned for her to work, and she ended up quitting.

I replaced Betty with Kathy, who was a nice step up as a do-all assistant, and I learned my second management lesson—don't ever feel like you are stuck with a marginal employee, because there is always somebody better out there to hire.

We gradually added staff as my practice grew to include a second office and an associate OD. I had eight non-OD staff members, as well as one employed OD when my practice was named in the top 2% in a nationwide survey conducted by the American Optometric Association in 1981.

About that time, my wife, Cris, and I converted a little 8' X 8' windowless room in our garage and started Hayes Marketing, Inc. to create customized recall cards, stationery, and patient education products for optometrists. Two years after that, we founded HMI Buying Group and moved into a real office. Once those two companies reached profitability, I gradually reduced my patient schedule and let my two associates take over. Unfortunately, I didn't have the benefit of my own future consulting advice, and had not structured my associates' compensation in a way that allowed the practice to be profitable unless I was there producing. That was yet another management mistake, and one of many lessons I learned early in my career.

As my businesses grew, I decided to sell my practice to my two associate ODs so I could devote all of my time helping other independent optometrists be more successful in their practices. I was only 38 and already retired from private practice, but my career as a business manager and team leader was just beginning.

The combined employee count at Hayes Marketing and HMI grew to over a hundred in the late 1980's, and nothing I studied in optometry school had prepared me to manage a company that big. In addition to on the job training, I learned how to manage by reading, taking courses, and working with great management consultants like Carl Hicks, Pat McMillan, and Jim Webb. Those three men deserve a lot of credit for helping me develop as business manager and team leader.

After 17 years in small town Mississippi, Cris and I decided we were ready for another business challenge, so we made the decision to move our family to Jacksonville, FL in 1990 and become an independent distributor for Vistakon. However, we didn't move the businesses—Hayes Marketing and HMI stayed in Vicksburg.

That's right, while I remained the CEO and owner, we turned over the operations of a company with one hundred employees and $10 million in annual sales to our management team, and moved to Florida. We were able to do that because we had created a sustainable business model that provided us with a high level of income and personal freedom, yet it did not require my input on a day-to-day basis.

Introduction

Dr. Neil Gailmard, my partner in Prima Eye Group, has done the same thing in his optometric practice and we now teach other high-producing ODs how to implement a model of practice that allows the owners to earn a higher income while enjoying more personal freedom as the practice grows.

Once we moved to Florida, I traveled back and forth to Mississippi every few months and that arrangement worked just fine until we decided to sell Hayes Marketing to Medical Arts Press in 1997. As of 2014, I still own HMI Buying Group and it's still based in Vicksburg.

I was in my late forties at the time we sold Hayes Marketing and retirement didn't appeal to me—so, with CibaVision™ as my lead investor, I started E-Dr., the first Internet based ordering platform for the optical industry. That company also grew to a hundred employees before it was downsized and sold in 2003. At that point, I had hired, fired, and made more mistakes with employees than most optometrists ever will.

I decided to put my management and financial experience to work for other optometrists, so I hired a sharp young MBA/CPA named Marilee Blackwell and started Hayes Consulting. Ms. Blackwell became a Certified Business Appraiser and we limited ourselves to practice valuations and profitability consulting for private practice ODs. Marilee was great at consulting, and was eventually able to take that business over and build a nice practice for herself.

The work I did at Hayes Consulting led to me being hired as the lead consultant for the practice finance portion of the Management & Business Academy started by Essilor™ and CibaVision™ in 2007. My company was responsible for gathering production data from the ODs who registered, as well as creating reports for the attendees. I would then give a two-hour lecture at every session on practice overhead and profitability. That lasted for about five years until Jobson Optical Research™ bought the program, and started doing the data gathering themselves.

I took a break until 2011 when I saw an opportunity to start a unique kind of consulting platform for optometrists with my now partner, Dr. Neil Gailmard. We created a new concept that incorporated his vast knowledge of practice management, and it went far beyond the narrow areas of practice finance and staff management I had worked in previously. That new firm is Prima Eye Group, and I have learned more about practice management from Neil and the high-producing ODs we work with over the last few years than I would have ever expected to.

Introduction

The hundreds of practices, big and small, I've worked with since starting Prima has given me a tremendous base of knowledge to write this book in an effort to share the information and experience I've gained over my career.

What my experience has taught me

I recently applied to join a Mastermind Group for business owners and one of the qualifying questions was *what is your 'unique ability?'* I've always struggled to answer that question because, false modesty aside, it was difficult for me to say what I'm really good at besides being creative, ambitious, and persistent.

For my own benefit, I gave the question some serious thought, and what I came to realize is that if I am good at anything in business, I am a team builder. I can recognize and attract talented people. I don't want to be the smartest guy in the room on every topic, and I actively seek to hire the brightest people I can find in their areas of expertise. I'm good at putting individuals of complementary strengths together, and directing them toward a common goal. I'm good at helping people grow on the job and perhaps, most importantly, I'm good at making sure my teams have the support they need to get good results.

How to Measure and Improve Staff Productivity

I certainly didn't start out this way in my optometric practice; but, as a result of being an absentee owner, I also became very good at delegating and allowing people to do their jobs without micromanaging the process. Delegation is something most optometrists could do more of, and later in the book we'll talk about why it's essential to be good at getting things done through others if you want to be a high producer.

Early in my business career, I realized there were many areas in which I lacked basic technical knowledge about the key daily operations that made the business run—marketing, design, and printing for Hayes Marketing, plus software and web development for E-Dr. What did I know about managing software engineers from India?

Coming out of a successful optometric practice, I had the mindset that I needed to know everything about every job and every process that went on in my office. I think many ODs want to do the same thing. That span of control approach worked during the start-up phase of Hayes Marketing, but the learning curve can be very steep when you have no background in areas like marketing, catalog production, and printing at Hayes Marketing and computer programing at E-Dr.

Fortunately, a wise consultant taught me early in my management career that I didn't have to know everything about every step of what went on in my

Introduction

companies. It was life-changing revelation to realize gradually that I could hire people smarter and more knowledgeable than I was, and let them do their jobs.

At this stage of my career, some might say I delegate too much and I could no doubt be better at monitoring my employees' work. But, I am good at mentoring and defining the results I want, and that's a big key to any success I have had. I believe in setting agreed upon outcomes for my staff and then letting them do the job to the best of their ability. Looking back, I know that has been a key secret to my success.

I decided to write this book because I have a passion for helping other optometrists become more successful, and the ODs I work with tell me I'm good at it.

Many of the management questions I get from optometrists revolve around three basic topics—how do I manage, compensate, and motivate my staff? I won't pretend to have all the answers; but, I wrote this book to share my opinions and teach you the process I use when consulting with other ODs.

Every situation is different. But, with some coaching and the basic knowledge provided on the following pages, every practice owner, big and small, can become even better at how to measure and improve team productivity.

How to Measure and Improve Staff Productivity

Enjoy the book, and feel free to email me with questions at jhayes@primaeyegroup.com.

How to use this book

The goal for providing you with this information is to teach practice owners not only some basic benchmarks and concepts, but also the philosophy behind my thinking so you can more effectively apply these ideas to your situation.

I want to be very clear that while I know from practical application the ideas in this book work, there is certainly more than one way to manage staff and be successful in private practice. So, feel free to use what you like, and discard the ideas that don't fit your personality.

Lastly, the book is written from the point of view of how we consult with the optometrists who belong to Prima Eye Group. However, you should know that my partner, Dr. Neil Gailmard, and I are like two chefs in the same kitchen in the sense that we don't use the same recipe to cook every meal. Our advice will almost always be similar, but rarely exactly the same. As I tell my staff when they hear different things from us—embrace the difference, and do what you think works best for you!

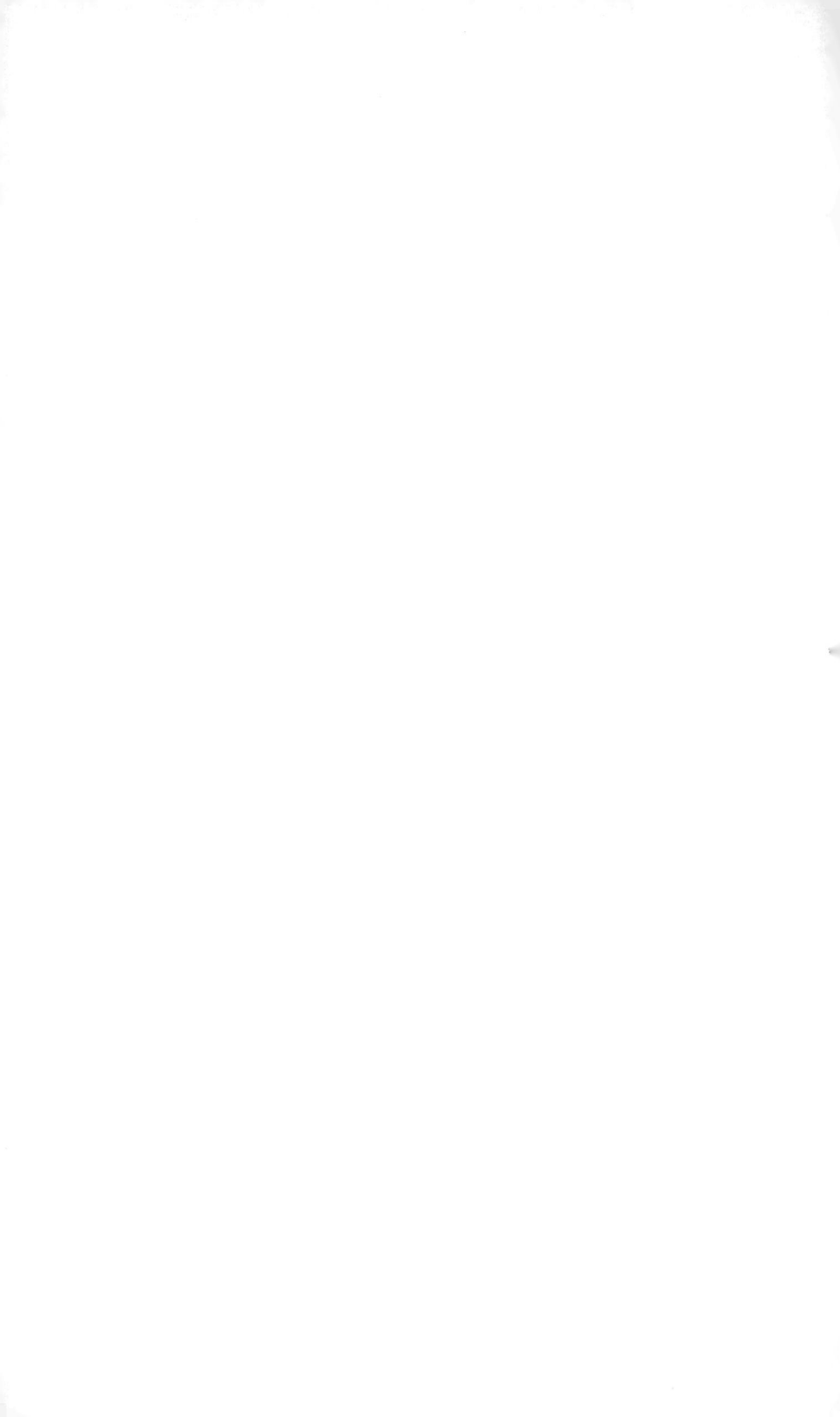

Chapter 1

What Are Your Obstacles to Growth?

Dear Jerry,

I have been in practice for over ten years, and I feel like I am stuck at $600,000 in annual gross income. I've tried a lot of things to increase my revenues, but we just can't seem to grow. What's your advice?

Ambitious in Arizona

What Are Your Obstacles to Growth

Before we get into a detailed discussion of team productivity, let's talk about some important metrics for overall practice production, and how they affect your ability to grow.

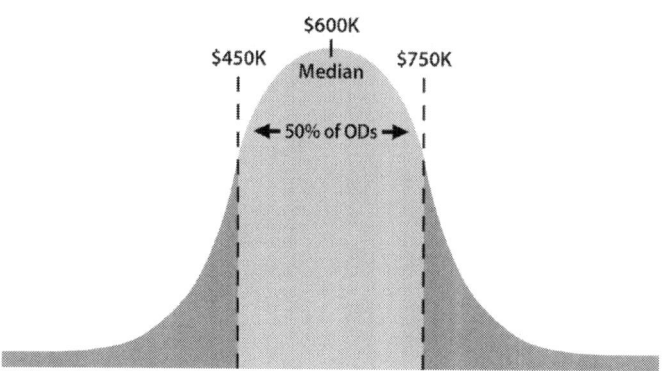

Fig. 1

According to surveys by the American Optometric Association, The Management & Business Academy Newsletter, and *Review of Optometry*, the median level of gross collected revenues per OD in private practice is approximately $600,000 per year. That's based on one FTE (full time equivalent) doctor working about 48 weeks on annual basis.

It's also worth noting that roughly 50% of all solo optometrists spend their entire careers in that

How to Measure and Improve Staff Productivity

$450,000 to $750,000 range of production. Most of the ODs I work with want to produce more than that, and I know they can. We'll use the rest of the book to discuss proven methods for improving your production and team productivity.

What are your obstacles to growth?

In my experience, all the things that keep an OD from seeing more patients and producing more income fall into five broad categories:

1. Doctor productivity
2. Staff productivity
3. Patient demand
4. Proper equipment
5. Office; location, capacity, and layout

When I ask optometrists at the $600,000 level of production what is holding them back, the default answer is always the same—lack of patient demand.

If that is really and truly your problem, we find the most overlooked aspect of patient demand is the role of customer service in retaining your existing patients and attracting new ones. My partner, Dr. Neil Gailmard, writes a lot about that, and it's a topic I will cover in detail in my next book *Success Secrets Of High Producing Optometrists*™.

This belief, right or wrong, is why most private practice ODs stay on an eternal search for practice marketing ideas. They think their problems will be solved if they can simply get more people to come in

What Are Your Obstacles to Growth

for appointments. However, as Dan Sullivan, CEO and Founder of Strategic Coach™ likes to say—the problem is never the problem.

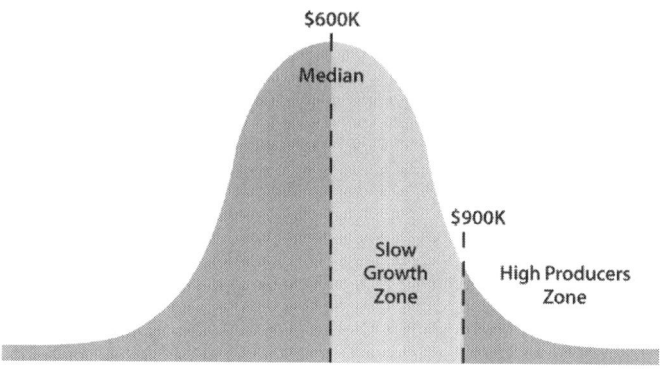

The slow growth zone is between $600,000 to $899,000

Fig. 2

The data tell us two things pretty clearly: 1) 50% of all ODs produce between $450,000 and $750,000 in annual revenues, and 2) there is a 'slow growth zone' that hits the average solo OD somewhere around $600,000 per year. Most practice owners who see their growth slow in this range will blame the same culprit we cited above (lack of patient demand) for their lack of growth.

Yet, I am curious why there always seems to be a million-dollar practice in the same town that is doing very well? Don't both optometrists have access to the

How to Measure and Improve Staff Productivity

same pool of potential patients who are coming in for eye care, as well as spending money on eyewear on a regular basis?

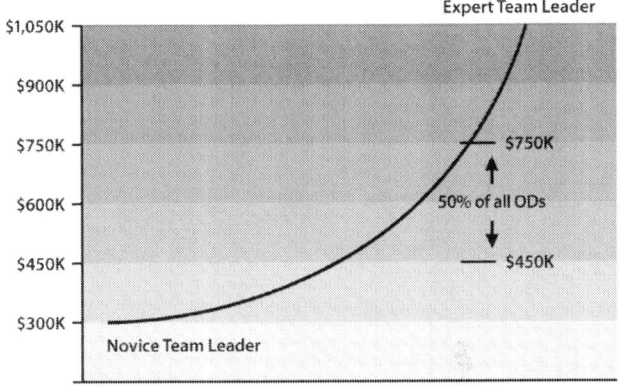

Fig. 3

Of course, there are many factors that go into how successful one practice is versus another. But, there is no doubt in my mind that the growth of a solo practice is directly related to the owner's level of management competence. And, it's no coincidence that this slow growth zone corresponds to the exact point at which an OD needs four or five employees to operate a practice.

Which leads me to one of the key conclusions of my thirty year practice management-consulting career—the first limiting factor to practice growth is an OD's ability to hire, manage, and lead an effective team of people. That limit may be a staff of two people for some docs, and a dozen for others.

What Are Your Obstacles to Growth

To be sure, there are other dynamics such as local competition, chair-side manner, the appearance of the office, ambition, and general business savvy that go into how much you gross. But, show me a practice that hasn't grown past $600,000 in gross revenues after four or five years, and I'll show you an OD who is struggling to manage a small team, and be a full time doctor at the same time. It's not easy.

Conversely, the OD who is grossing $900,000 solo and netting 30% with six full time employees is doing a lot of things right in terms of leveraging his production through a well-trained staff. My conclusion is that the optometrists who have been able to break through that slow growth barrier are the ones who are good delegators by virtue of training, prior experience, or just innate leadership skills.

The good news and the reason for writing this book, is that there are proven ways practice owners can improve their skills as team leaders.

How long is your appointment backlog?

One of the simple metrics I use to assess patient demand is asking optometrists how long their appointment backlog is. Whenever that question comes up, I am reminded of a conversation with Dr. Steven Weisfeld of New Jersey who produced $1.2

How to Measure and Improve Staff Productivity

Million as a solo OD in 2013. That's double the national average.

When I asked Steve how far in advance he was scheduled, he answered, "What backlog? I am typically booked out no more than a day or two. My philosophy is to get people in as fast as I can." That's great advice from one of the highest producing solo ODs with whom I have ever consulted.

We talk to optometrists in $600,000 practices all the time who claim to be booked up two to three weeks in advance. A long waiting time for an appointment in a practice that size—say more than one or two weeks—tells me the doctor is either not productive enough, or that he is greatly underutilizing his staff. These doctors don't have a problem with patient demand—they just need to see the ones they have now in a more timely fashion.

If you are one of the those fortunate optometrists who is consistently booked up more than a few days in advance, that is the same as having people standing in line waiting to give you money. If revenue growth is your objective, don't make people wait any longer than absolutely necessary to see you. Do what Dr. Weisfeld does, collapse that backlog and get those patients in as fast as you can. Making patients wait weeks for an appointment is bad business when you're a private practice optometrist. Getting those people in faster

What Are Your Obstacles to Growth

for their appointments will feed on itself, and become a big practice builder for you.

How many patients can you see in a day?

According to the Management & Business Academy, private practice optometrists producing over $750,000 per year see an average of 1.5 patients per hour. That equates to 60 patients in a 40 hour week (1.5 X 40).

60 patients X $300 per exam = $18,000 per week

$18,000 X 50 weeks = $900,000 per year

At the other end of the spectrum, ODs producing less than $500,000 per year see an average of .76 patients per hour, or about 30 per week (.76 X 40).

30 patients X $300 per exam = $9,000 per week

$9,000 X 50 weeks = $450,000 per year

If you are producing $600,000 to $750,000 and booked up more than a week in advance on a consistent basis, that tells us that patient demand is not the problem you might think it is. It's one of the other four items on our list;

2. Doctor capacity
3. Staff capacity
4. Proper equipment
5. Office—location, capacity, and layout

A newer, nicer office is a practice builder

Now, what about items 4 and 5, your office space and equipment? The thing that keeps many ODs from producing more is that their office, equipment, and staff are geared around seeing 40, not 60, patients a week. In other words, most ODs don't practice in offices that are designed to gross $1,000,000 a year, even when the demand is there.

But, Jerry, optometrists often tell me, *my office is too small, I only have one exam room, we have a poor location, there is no room to expand,* and the list goes on. These are all valid reasons they can't see more patients and, if that's the case, my advice to any growth minded ODs is—do something about it.

You can't tell the fire, "Give me some heat, and then I'll throw on the wood." Be smart about how much you spend and don't overdo it; but, if you stay booked up more than a week in advance and you sense the demand building in your practice, I say, "Build it because they are already there!"

If enhanced customer service is the number one under-appreciated way to build patient demand, a new office is certainly number two on the list. I don't have hard data, but reliable reports over the years from doctors—and, suppliers like EyeDesigns™ who sell to them—moving into nicer, bigger office space in a good location usually results in an increase of gross income of 25% within two years. It happened for me years ago, and every OD I have worked with reports the same bump in revenues when they upgrade their office. Dr. Gailmard has told me more than once that having a nice, big, well-located office is an essential key to his success.

How do you know if investing time and money to expand your office will pay off? Your business advisor or the consultants at Prima Eye Group can do a breakeven analysis for you that will determine how much you can invest in a new office without spending too much. For example, let's say you are typically booked up one week in advance and that you see an average of 10 exams per day, four days per week. That comes out to 40 per week X $300 = $12,000.

If you reduce that backlog and see two more patients per day, that will increase your exams from 40 to 48 per week and your revenues from $12,000 per week to $14,400.

That extra $2,400 per will week increase your annual revenues from $576,000 (48 weeks X $12,000) to $691,200 (48 X $12,000). An increase of $115,200!

At 30% net, that extra revenue will increase your pre-tax practice profits from $172,800 (30% X $576,000) to $207,360 (30% X $691,200). That's almost $35,000 in extra profits.

How to Measure and Improve Staff Productivity

Depending on how much you need to invest in a new office or equipment—if any—your net percent may actually increase slightly as your revenues rise because your fixed overhead will stay the same while your staff and cost of goods will increase at the same ratios as your revenues.

Chapter highlights:

1. The first limiting factor to practice growth is an OD's ability to hire, manage, and lead an effective team of people.
2. The slow growth zone for the majority of ODs occurs somewhere between $600,000 and $750,000 in gross collected revenues.
3. A long waiting time for an appointment in a practice grossing $600,000 suggests the doctor is not productive enough, or he is underutilizing his staff.

Chapter 2

Doctor Productivity

Dear Jerry,

I gross $600,000 a year solo, and I'm having trouble breaking through to the next level. Is it really possible for one OD to gross $1 million or more in private practice? If so, what does it take to do that?

Working Hard in Washington

Doctor Productivity

Yes, I've personally worked with a number of solo optometrists who are individually producing a million dollars or more in private practice. Needless to say, you can't do that without a great team, and we're to going give you many good ideas on how to develop one in the next nine chapters.

If you're currently working hard to build a dream practice and improve your own production, let me share a little story about how self-imposed limits keep many intelligent and hard-working people from achieving their maximum professional and personal success.

In 1945, the world record time for running the mile was set at 4:01.3. That time, just over four minutes, stood for nine long years, without being lowered by even one millisecond.

Why? A big reason was that all the world-class athletes and medical experts of the day truly believed that the human body was not physically capable of running a sub four-minute mile.

That thinking was changed forever on May 6, 1954, when Roger Bannister, a young British medical student, ran the mile in a record-breaking time of 3:59.4.

How to Measure and Improve Staff Productivity

It was an historic feat to be sure. But what followed was equally remarkable. The four-minute threshold, a barrier that was largely considered unobtainable, was suddenly broken over a dozen times in a matter of months by a variety of runners. A coincidence?

Not at all. Once Sir Roger, now a highly regarded neurologist in London, showed the other competitors who trained just as hard as he that a man could run a four-minute mile, the psychological barriers were lifted. Their belief was completely changed because, as soon as these other talented runners saw someone else run a sub four-minute mile, they KNEW they could too.

How does this true story apply to you? Many well trained, highly intelligent and perfectly capable OD's are held back from greater satisfaction and financial success in private practice not by competition, lack of patient demand or even low paying third party plans.

They are held back for no other reason than they don't believe they, or any other OD, can really produce $1 million or more individually in private practice.

Figuring out how to grow your practice to the next level—whether your goal is $600,000 or $1,600,000—is a lot like running a four-minute mile. Once you know it can be done, a seemingly unattainable goal suddenly becomes very, very doable. Now it's just a question of how.

But, before we get into a detailed analysis of staff productivity, let's talk about some important metrics for overall practice production.

What it takes to produce $600,000

Let's look at two key variables: 1) the number of exams performed, and 2) revenue per comprehensive examination to see what it takes for an optometrist actually to produce the median level of $600,000 in gross collected revenue per year.

According to the American Optometric Association and the Management & Business Academy, the median revenue per comprehensive examination for private practice ODs is a little over $300. This figure is calculated by dividing your total practice income by the number of 'comprehensive examinations' performed in one year. Example:

$600,000 gross revenue ÷ 2,000 exams = $300

Therefore, a solo OD averaging $300 per comprehensive examination will have to perform 2,000 exams to gross $600,000.

A few notes on this calculation—because your total collected gross revenues will always include some income from medical visits and progress checks other than comprehensive exams, we know that

How to Measure and Improve Staff Productivity

'revenue per exam' is one of those practice management calculations that will never be exact. But, that's OK because this is a benchmarking exercise that doesn't require the same accuracy as balancing your checkbook or doing your tax return.

The point is, don't let the lack of precision drive you crazy or keep you from tracking this extremely important metric. Once you start monitoring revenue per exam, you will figure out ways to make it grow.

We also realize the definition of 'comprehensive exam' will vary from practice to practice—our definition is an exam with a refraction. No matter how you define it, the key to making this a meaningful number for your practice is to be consistent with how you calculate it on a year-to-year basis in your office.

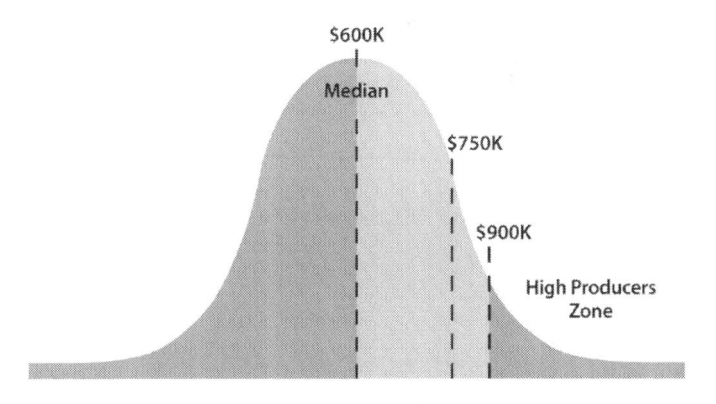

Fig. 4

Only 25% of ODs produce more than $750,000

Doctor Productivity

What it takes to produce $1,000,000

I asked the OD who used to be in charge of practice surveys for the American Optometric Association, Dr. Richard Edlow, for his input on what percentage of optometrists are high producers. Based on the data we both reviewed, our best estimate is that about 20 - 25% of private practice ODs produce more than $750,000 per year, and only 10% produce more than $900,000 per year. Again, that's per doctor, not per practice.

Which means the percent of ODs individually producing over $1,000,000 in private practice is pretty small. I would estimate it's no more than 5%, maybe less.

Yet, the math works exactly the same for high producing ODs as it does for those in medium-sized practices. If an optometrist averages $300 per comprehensive examination, that means the doctor has to do 3,333 exams per year to produce $1,000,000 in gross revenue.

$1,000,000 gross revenue ÷ $3,333 exams = $300

At 50 weeks per year, a doctor will need to perform an average of 67 comprehensive examinations per week to achieve a total of 3,333 in one year.

66.6 exams X 50 weeks = 3,330 exams

67 exams ÷ 5 = 13.4 exams per day

How to Measure and Improve Staff Productivity

Thirteen to fourteen exams per day may seem like a lot if you are grossing $600,000 per year. But we consult with many ODs who routinely perform fifteen to twenty exams per day. We're not face-to-face, but I know what you are thinking—*I don't have the demand to book 67 patients a week for comprehensive exams*. I realize that patient demand is a major challenge for many optometrists. But, don't dismiss that level of production as unachievable. It doesn't happen overnight for anybody, but it is something that you can grow into over time.

Revenue per comprehensive exam

It's also important to keep in mind that the number of exams performed is only one variable in a two part equation. Average revenue per exam is the second variable that will greatly affect the total gross income you can produce and collect. For example, what if your average revenue per exam were $500 instead of $300?

$500 X 2,000 exams = $1,000,000 gross revenue

2,000 exams ÷ 50 weeks = 40 exams per week

As the numbers show, a doctor producing $600,000 per year can see the same number of patients and raise their production to $1,000,000 per year 'simply' by increasing their revenue per exam from $300 to $500.

Doctor Productivity

Is it possible to raise your revenue per exam over time? Of course it is, and there are a number of ways to do that. The highest revenue number we currently work with is Dr. Warren Johnson and his wife Kay who average $850 per comprehensive exam in their Memphis office. Only to say, there is a lot of room to grow your revenues on a per patient basis above the national average of $300. Having said that, most of the ODs we work with and are producing $1,000,000 a year are averaging closer to $400 or $500 per exam, not $850.

Chapter highlights:

1. The median production per private practice OD is $600,000 per year.
2. 50% of all ODs spend their careers producing somewhere between $450,000 and $750,000 in collected gross revenues.
3. The two variables affecting practice production are the number of exams seen per year, and the average revenue per exam.

Chapter 3

How Big Does My Team Need to Be?

Dear Jerry,

Some members of my staff complain that they are too busy, and we need to hire another person. I'm not sure I agree. How do I know the right number of non-OD employees for a practice my size?

Thanks for your help,

Busy in Birmingham

How Big Does My Team Need to Be?

Archimedes famously said, "Give me a lever and a place which to put a fulcrum, and I can move the world."

That statement is extremely apropos to private practice optometrists because the number of patients you see, as well as the amount of dollars you generate will always be directly related to how well you leverage the productivity of your staff. The more you delegate to your staff, the more patients you should be able to see on a per doctor basis.

How much should you delegate?

How much should you delegate in terms of patient care and office management? The answer depends on what you are comfortable with. I'm a patient of a busy retinal specialist at Mayo Clinic in Jacksonville, FL where the technician does visual fields, Goldmann tonometry, and what I find to be a very good refraction. 'All' the doctor does is the ophthalmoscopy and case presentation. What I've come to realize from talking to many ophthalmologists is that they are comfortable with delegation because that's the way they've been trained.

It's unfortunate that we don't get more training in optometry school on how to use technicians because my experience is that vast majority of optometrists could reduce stress, work less, make

How to Measure and Improve Staff Productivity

more, and provide a higher level of care—all good objectives—if we learned to delegate more to well trained staff. Fortunately, delegation is a pretty easy thing to learn on your own once you get over the idea that you don't have to do everything yourself for patients to be satisfied with your service.

Which begs the question, how far down the road of delegating do you want to go? I've consulted with ODs who still write up their own lab orders and dispense glasses because they feel they can do it better than their staff. And, they probably can. But, that is a terribly inefficient way to practice.

As we said in Chapter 1, the median gross revenue for a dispensing optometrist is $600,000 per year. Of that $600,000, only 37% is produced directly by the one thing that relies on the doctor—exams. The implication, of course, is that your staff should be the primary producer of the other 63% of revenue produced in your practice.

Source Of OD Income

- Professional Fees   37%
- Contacts   17%
- Frames   18%
- Spectacle Lenses   27%

Source: Howard Purcell, O.D., F.A.A.O., Dipl.
Senior VP of Customer Development
Essilor of America, Inc.

Fig. 5

How Big Does My Team Need to Be?

Many solo ODs tell me they are very busy and want to delegate more, but they fear they will lose the patients who want to see only them. I jokingly tell them that I am a patient at Mayo Clinic—$8 billion in annual revenues—and I've never seen Dr. Mayo even once.

Some optometrists I work with have delegated patient care to the point that their staff and employed ODs manage the day-to-day operations of the practice without the owner being present. Dr. Neil Gailmard and his wife, Dr. Susan Gailmard, have built a multimillion-dollar practice that runs so well they are able to take off extended periods of time. Employed associate ODs see the vast majority of patients at Gailmard Eye Center, and their practice just keeps growing.

For those of you who think this causes the quality of patient care to suffer, the answer is—not that I can see. I know a number of other ODs who delegate the majority of patient care in great practices that provide a high level of care and produce a nice income for the owner.

The point is when done properly, delegating should increase, not decrease quality of care, revenues, and profits. It's also an important part of the answer to how you stay profitable in this age of managed care, vision plans, and reduced fees.

How big does my team need to be?

Staffing levels for your practice will vary depending on a number of factors such as:

1. Collected gross revenues
2. Revenue per patient
3. Office layout and equipment
4. Doctor's willingness to delegate patient care as well as management duties
5. Leadership and systems—how well your team is trained and organized

Based on my analysis of staffing levels in hundreds of both high producing and low producing private practices, we know that a good range for non-OD team productivity is between $125,000 and $175,000 in revenue per FTE per year.

Revenue per employee is calculated by simply dividing your annual collected gross income by the number of all your non-OD employees.

Example; $900,000 ÷ 6 FTE staff = $150,000.

Note: one FTE (fulltime equivalent employee) means that person works approximately forty hours per week, and forty-eight to fifty weeks per year. In the event you have part time employees, you should compute a fractional amount. For example, someone working twenty hours per week equals .5 FTE. Two part time employees working twenty hours per week equals one FTE (2 employees X 20 hours per week = 40 hours).

You should include all your clerical staff such as bookkeepers and insurance clerks in this calculation as they are essential to the everyday operations of your practice.

If you have a multimillion dollar practice with a big optical staff for edging or surfacing, you might want to leave your bench opticians out of this calculation. The theory is that if you sent all your jobs to an outside lab, you wouldn't be employing all those people. Otherwise, just count everybody on your payroll.

How to analyze team productivity

We analyze team productivity in an optometric practice based on the dollars produced per employee per annum. At the beginning of 2014, the median for non-OD team productivity among over 200 practices that we actually analyzed in detail was $153,000 per employee per year. The highest level of staff productivity in this group of practices in Prima Eye Group was $285,000 and the lowest level was $94,000.

To get an idea of why this number can vary so much, let's look at three separate solo practices with annual gross collected revenues of $900,000. One practice has nine FTEs, one has six, and one has four.

Annual production per team member
Practice 1: $900,000 gross ÷ 9 FTE = $100,000
Practice 2: $900,000 gross ÷ 6 FTE = $150,000
Practice 3: $900,000 gross ÷ 4 FTE = $225,000

We are sometimes asked if we track revenue on a per employee basis, and the answer for this analysis is no. Some doctors like to track individual sales in the dispensary; but, in this analysis, the only number we are worried about is the average of dollars produced per employee in the whole practice.

A comfortable level of team productivity

In the case of practice 2 above, six non-OD FTEs producing an average of $150,000 will result in gross collected revenues of $900,000.

$900,000 gross ÷ 6 employees = $150,000

A production level of $150,000 per FTE, per year, puts practice 2 very comfortably in the middle of my recommended range.

Low team productivity

Practice 1 has $900,000 in gross collected revenues, and nine non-OD FTE staff members.

$900,000 gross ÷ 9 FTEs = $100,000

I consider a productivity level of $100,000 per employee, per year, to be low for a traditional dispensing optometric practice. This tells me the practice is slightly over staffed.

There are usually three causes for low team productivity. One, the practice owner doesn't know how to measure productivity or evaluate it based on revenues. So, when the staff complains that they are too busy, he takes the path of least resistant and hires another person. Do this a few times and you end up with more people than you need for the work to be done.

Two, a low producing staff tells me the practice owner needs to get more organized in terms of job descriptions, who does what, and setting clear production goals for his practice. If this is your situation, you may need a full time office manager or possibly spend more time on management yourself. We'll talk about that in the next chapter.

A third possible cause of low team productivity is a low level of revenue on a per patient basis. This can be due to low fees or a low capture rate in your dispensary. Example:

As we said above, the median dispensing practice generates about $300 per comprehensive exam. Which means the median OD has to see 2,000

How to Measure and Improve Staff Productivity

exams per year, or 40 exams per week, to produce $600,000 in a year.

$600,000 ÷ $300 = 2,000 exams per year
2,000 exams ÷ 50 weeks = 40 exams per week

But, what if a practice averages only $200 per exam? That OD has to see 4,500 exams per year or 90 exams per week to produce the same $900,000.

$600,000 ÷ $200 = 3,000 exams per year
3,000 exams ÷ 50 weeks = 60 exams per week

As the math tells us, the owner of a low fee practice has to do more exams to produce the same amount of gross revenue as a medium or high fee practice owner. That's why revenue per patient has a direct impact on how much staff a practice needs.

In my experience, very low team productivity is a case where the practice owner needs to evaluate both her overall fees on private pay sales and the dispensing capture rate of patients seen for eye examinations.

High team productivity—it's not a good thing!

Now, let's look at a scenario where an OD with a $900,000 gross revenue practice has only four non-OD team members, and what I consider to be a high productivity per staff number.

$900,000 ÷ 4 employees = $225,000

How Big Does My Team Need to Be?

Like the citizens of Garrison Keillor's Lake Wobegon, we all want to be above average. This, however, is a case where more is not better. In my experience, anything over $175,000 in productivity per non-OD employee means the practice may be understaffed. There are usually three causes when the staff productivity number gets this high: one, the doctor is very efficient, and ends up doing many of the staff functions herself. That is another way of saying she is not delegating enough of the patient care and management duties. This is very common in practices grossing under $600,000. Yes, doctors who spend a lot of time helping with the busy work of their practice might save some money by not hiring an extra person. But, that usually means they aren't devoting enough time playing the role of CEO and thinking about how to take their practice to the next level.

Two, it's a well-organized team producing close to their maximum. We see many hard working, high producing, practice owners who fall in this trap. The problem is practice growth will stagnate when the staff is pushed to maximum level of productivity. You don't want to buy clothes for a growing baby that fit just right—you want to allow some room for them to get bigger. It's the same logic for your team—you need to overstaff slightly for peak times, or your production will plateau.

How to Measure and Improve Staff Productivity

We usually see production and growth max out when a practice hits the $175,000 to $200,000 per staff range. In most cases, a level of productivity that high is a clear signal that you need to hire another person if you want your practice to continue to grow. My advice to ODs in this situation is don't think about the $35,000 a new employee is going to cost—think about the extra $140,000 they are going to help you produce. That's a 4:1 return on investment!

Three, in some cases high team productivity can be the result of a high fee practice that generates well above the average revenue per exam. In this event, $200,000 in FTE productivity per year could possibly be a good thing! Example:

As we saw above, the average practice grossing $600,000 does about $300 per comprehensive exam and sees 2,000 exams per year. That works out to 40 exams per week.

$600,000 ÷ $300 = 2,000 exams per year
2,000 exams ÷ 50 weeks = 40 exams per week

Now let's compare that to a higher fee practice that averages $600 per patient. That means this OD needs to see only 1,000 exams per year, or 20 exams per week, to gross $600,000. That, of course, is HALF of the number of patients our low practice owner has to see.

$600,000 ÷ $600 = 1,000 exams per year
1,000 exams ÷ 50 weeks = 20 exams per week

How Big Does My Team Need to Be?

It stands to reason an optometrist seeing 1,000 exams per year will need fewer employees than one seeing 2,000 exams per year.

The math suggests that high fee practices will have much higher than average team productivity; that, too, varies in the real world.

The two highest fee practices in terms of revenue per comprehensive exam I worked with recently fell very much in the normal range for team productivity.

As I said earlier, Dr. Warren Johnson and his wife Kay, who is the office manager, average over $850 per patient in their Memphis, TN practice, which is the highest number we have seen. But, his staff productivity is right in line at $132,000 per employee per year. That suggests to me that his staff spends a lot of time with their patients.

Drs. Jeff and Kristy Frank of Spex Expressions in Sycamore, IL average an impressive $650 per comprehensive exam in their practice while their team productivity is $170,000 per FTE per year. That's a little high, but well in line with our recommended ranges, especially given their above average revenues per exam.

On the other hand, Dr. Todd Cohan of Forsight Vision in nearby Long Grove, IL averages the same $650 per comprehensive exam as the

How to Measure and Improve Staff Productivity

Franks, but his staff productivity number is high at $264,000 per FTE. He is the exception that makes the rule.

The point is even practices with very high revenue per exams numbers still have normal ranges for their productivity per staff.

Chapter highlights:
1. Your staff is the lever for increasing your productivity as a doctor. The way to increase production is delegate as much as you practically can.
2. How much staff you need is a function of your annual practice revenues.
3. A comfortable level of production is $150,000 per non-OD staff per year. Anything under $125,000 is too low while production over $175,000 is a sign that you may be understaffed for future growth.

Chapter 4

When Do You Need an Office Manager?

Dear Jerry,

My solo practice had $600,000 in gross collected revenues last year, and I have three full time employees plus two part timers for a total of five. Do you think it's time for me to appoint or hire an office manager to take some the administrative and management load off of myself? What's the magic number?

Managing in Maryland

When Do You Need an Office Manager?

The answer is every practice needs an office manager from day one. In a small practice with one, two, or three employees that role is almost always filled by the doctor/owner. That's certainly the way it was during the beginning stages of my practice. But, if I have to pick a point at which most ODs need to actually designate an office manager, it would be when your gross collected revenues hit that slow growth stage at around $600,000 per year in revenues.

I use $600,000 as my benchmark because I think most ODs can see all the patients, oversee the administration, and manage three or four employees by themselves in a practice producing $599,000 or less. But, once your production exceeds the $600,000 level and requires four or five employees, a paralyzing level of complexity sets in that slows the growth of 75% of all private practices.

As you already know, getting busier with patients creates a ripple effect in other areas of your office which, in turn, creates more demands on your time as depicted in the accompanying illustration. What you can't see and readily measure for yourself is that practice growth slows about the time you max out in your ability to effectively manage the clinical, staff, financial, and customer service components of your practice. And, that is why I think so many ODs get

How to Measure and Improve Staff Productivity

stuck there—it is extremely difficult to diagnose being the neck in one's own bottle.

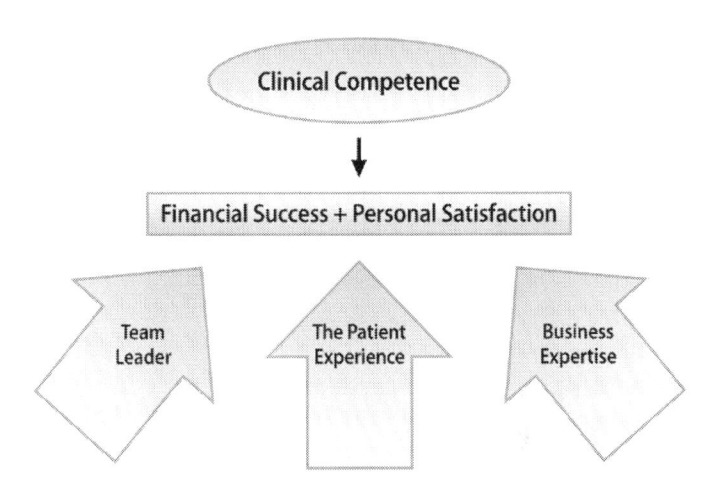

```
          Clinical Competence
                  ↓
   Financial Success + Personal Satisfaction
     ↑              ↑              ↑
   Team         The Patient     Business
   Leader       Experience      Expertise
```

Four roles an OD must fill to succeed in private practice

Fig. 6

What we're trying to communicate in this graphic is that there are four essential roles that every practice owner must fill if he or she is going to be financially successful in private practice. They are:

1. Full time clinician
2. Team leader
3. Business administrator
4. Head of customer service

Since 99% of our training is patient oriented, doctors have a natural tendency to focus the majority of our time and efforts on clinical duties. But, you're not going to successfully compete with ophthalmology and corporate eye care, and stay

How Much Should I Pay My Staff?

profitable unless somebody fills those roles. The good news is that somebody doesn't have to be you.

So, as you get busier seeing patients when your practice grows, the rest of the workload, along with the complexity, increases proportionally in all four areas. Here is what I mean:

$300,000 revenue practice

If a practice averages $300 per complete exam and sees 1,000 exams per year, gross revenues should be about $300,000 ($300 X 1,000 exams). That will require two non-OD employees at an average of $150,000 per staff ($300,000 ÷ 2 = $150,000).

So, in addition to your duties as doctor, business administrator, and head of customer service you also have to manage two full time employees. That should be pretty easy for any OD who wants to make a go of it in private practice.

$600,000 revenue practice

In order for the same doctor to gross $600,000 at an average of $300 per complete exam, he will have to see 2,000 patients per year ($300 X 2,000 exams).

That will typically require four non-OD employees at an average of $150,000 per staff ($600,000 ÷ 4 = $150,000).

How to Measure and Improve Staff Productivity

Which means he now has to oversee four full time employees plus his other three duties. In many cases, he'll have a couple of part timers splitting one of those full time positions, so this doctor is probably managing five employees. And, of course, each employee takes pretty much the same amount of time and energy to manage whether they are part time or full time.

$900,000 revenue practice

To gross $900,000 at an average of $300 per complete exam, he will have to see 3,000 exams per year ($300 X 3,000 exams).

That will require six non-OD FTEs at an average of $150,000 per full time staff ($900,000 ÷ 6 = $150,000). Which means he is now managing eight or nine employees plus the increased workload in the clinical, customer service, and business areas.

So, whether it's $450,000, $750,000 or somewhere in between, you need to designate an effective office manager the moment you sense you need help, or you're never going to make it to the top 10% of ODs who gross $900,000.

Three ways to hire an office manager

Private practice optometry is a team sport, and building a great staff is absolutely essential for ODs who want to keep growing. Once you feel that practice growth is slowing, or that the everyday management is getting more complex than you can comfortably handle by yourself, it's already past time

How Much Should I Pay My Staff?

to consider designating an office manager. If you're grossing near that $600,000 mark and starting to wonder if you need a strong office manager, the answer is probably yes. Here are three ways to fill that role in your practice:

One, you can groom one of your current employees for this key position. That assumes you already have the right person on your staff as this is not the position for a social promotion for good behavior and longevity in your office. This will be one of the most important hires you ever make in terms of the future success of your practice.

A common mistake we see is for an OD to promote a strong bookkeeper or optician into the office manager role knowing they having glaring weakness such as managing people. My strong advice is don't designate an existing employee with a limited skill set to be your OM just to fill the role. Otherwise, the management duties they can't perform will continue to fall on your shoulders.

Two, if you don't have the right person on staff, you may need to hire someone from the outside. I did this when I hired a sales rep from my local office supply company, and that worked out extremely well for me. Of course, there is always a concern that the existing staff might resent being passed over for a promotion, even if no one is deserving. You can take some of the mystery out of this process by interviewing and testing members of your own staff.

Three, you can reduce or compress your own appointment schedule to cut back on one or more of your patient days, and spend more time as CEO of your own practice. I did this as my practice grew and Dr. Neil Gailmard has raised the CEO role to an art form in his multimillion-dollar practice. Any OD with a reasonable interest in practice management can do a great job if they are willing to get support and learn from others.

If you're busy enough to consider being your own office manager, this would be a good time to have a trusted financial advisor or the consultants at Prima run a feasibility analysis on whether or not you can afford an employed OD to see patients and give you some free time to manage the practice.

Four traits of a great office manager

Whether you are approaching $600,000 in production, or you're well past that level and you just need to build management depth on your staff, here are the four key attributes I suggest you look for in an office manager or practice administrator. Prima offers an excellent series of pre employment personal assessments to help you identify these traits.

1. The ability to manage people. In an ideal world, all of your staff would report not to you, but your office manager. This would relieve you of having

to deal with multiple people problems on a daily basis.

A good office manager should be able to handle staff work schedules, answer operational questions and serve as a buffer between you and the staff.

2. The ability to manage your practice overhead. A surprising number of optometrists spend very little time monitoring their overhead expenses. This tells me they are missing a golden opportunity to increase practice profitability.

If you happen to be one of those ODs who hate the business side of practice, that's OK as you have plenty of company. Nobody is going to care as much about the success of your practice as you do, but good consultants can add a lot in terms of oversight and training in this area for you, and your staff.

3. The ability to operate independently. A good office manager should not have to come to you every time an operational decision has to be made. Some ODs don't like to delegate, but every management duty you are willing to hand off frees you up to take time off, or play the CEO role. It takes a while to mentor someone in that position plus a willingness on your part to delegate. What are you waiting for?

4. The ability to get results. For me, the Holy Grail is to find a manager who is achievement oriented. Once you set goals for your practice, this is

How to Measure and Improve Staff Productivity

a person with the innate ability to get things done without you having to direct their every move. This may sound far fetched if you don't have a strong 'can do' person on your staff now. But, I know they are out there because we consult with very capable office managers on a regular basis. It's a thing of beauty when you get one.

What about million dollar practices?

Reminder: if you're in a group practice, that $600,000 becomes a multiple of the Full Time Equivalent doctors in your practice. That's $1,200,000 for two doctors, $1,800,000 for three doctors and so on.

The problem I often see in bigger practices is that while the gross revenues have grown nicely above the million-dollar level, the OD owner continues to hire lower level staff when she really needs to start developing one or two employees that can help in a management capacity. Otherwise, she will remain locked into the role of de facto office manager whether she likes it or not. Common symptoms of having too many followers and not enough leaders are:

1. Every staff member is a direct report to the doctor.
2. No one on the staff has an official leadership role. I say 'official' because every staff has leaders whether designated by the practice owner or not.

3. The doctor feels that every day-to-day decision winds up on her desk whether she wants it or not.
4. The doctor feels tied to the practice and is hesitant to take time off or go on vacation because they are afraid things will fall apart.

That's the bad news. The good news is that if you're willing to hire and train the right people, and then delegate more of the day-to-day management activities in your practice, your life in the office can become a lot more fun.

The trick to becoming a good CEO of your own practice is to create the right management structure, and then put the right people in place.

Chapter highlights:

1. Every practice needs an office manager from day one.
2. Once your production exceeds the $600,000 level and requires four or five employees, a level of complexity sets in that slows the growth of 75% of all private practices.
3. There are three ways to fill the role of office manager: 1) promote from within, 2) hire from the outside, and 3) become your own CEO.

Chapter 5

How Much Should I Pay My Staff?

Dear Jerry,

I want to know how much I should be paying my non-OD staff. I have a 30% net practice, but my staff expenses seem out of line at 25% of total practice revenues. Is that something I should be concerned about?

Thanks for your help,

Overpaying in Oregon

How Much Should I Pay My Staff?

Let's start this chapter by defining what goes into the staff expense category. Basically, it's everything you pay your staff such as: salaries, FICA, bonuses, health insurance, retirement programs, travel, training, and uniforms. If you spend something on your team, the person who does your bookkeeping should allocate that expenditure to staff.

One mistake we see fairly often is for the bookkeeper or accountant to lump non-OD staff expenses together with what practice owners pay their employed associate ODs. That's not a good idea because it distorts practice overhead, and makes it difficult for you and us to do a good production analysis. Therefore, the salary you pay employed ODs or partner ODs should be allocated to a different category than what you pay your non-OD staff.

For most optometrists, staff is the second biggest overhead category after cost of goods. However, I encourage you to think of your team as an investment, not an expense. As we said in the previous chapter, your practice should be producing somewhere around $150,000 per team member, so every time you add a full time employee, your revenues should increase by roughly that amount until you're ready to hire the next employee.

How to Measure and Improve Staff Productivity

In terms of the percent of gross you should spend on staff, there is no magic number—such as 20%—that applies to every practice. That's because over the last the two decades, the revenues optometrists produce from medical visits have increased and the proportional amount we spend on optical lab bills has decreased due to vision plans.

Those gradual changes in income and expense have caused us to analyze optometric overhead in a slightly different way. Now, instead of looking at just your staff expense, we want to know the total of your Cost of Goods plus your staff costs as a percent of your overall practice revenues.

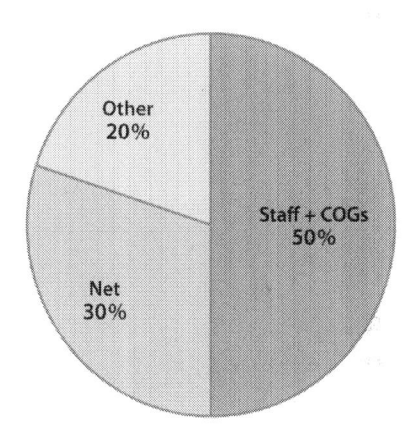

Other 20%
Staff + COGs 50%
Net 30%

Key financial indicators for private practice optometrists

Fig. 7

As you can see from the pie chart above, if you want to net the national average of 30%, the combination of your staff salaries and cost of goods

How Much Should I Pay My Staff?

should not exceed 50% of your total gross collected revenues.

So, to answer the question of how much you should spend on staff, I really don't care whether your mix is 30% COGS/ 20% staff, or 25% COGS/ 25% staff, as long as the combination of your staff's salaries plus your cost of goods does not exceed the magic 50%.

To illustrate why, let's look at the overhead of a typical 30% net practice in which the staff salaries and COGS are both 25% of collected gross revenues.

Collected Gross Income		$1,000,000
COGS	25%	250,000
Staff	25%	250,000
Fixed Overhead	20%	200,000
Total Expenses	70%	700,000
Practice Net	30%	300,000

Simple math tells us that if you want to net the national average of 30% of gross revenues and your fixed overhead consisting of rent, utilities, marketing, equipment, and general office overhead is 20% of gross, the sum of your staff expenses and COGS cannot exceed the other 50% of revenues.

Here are three more examples of how staff costs and cost of goods go together to impact your practice overhead:

Example 1, average costs—good ratio

Cost of goods   30%
Staff   20%

Good ratio = 50%

Example 2, high staff costs—good ratio

Cost of goods   23%
Staff   27%

Good ratio = 50%

Example 3, high staff costs—bad ratio

Cost of goods   35%
Staff   25%

Bad ratio = 60%

These ratios help you understand why it's imperative to take a big picture view of your practice

How Much Should I Pay My Staff?

overhead before you decide to raise an existing team member's pay, or make an offer to a promising new employee. You need to look at each individual's compensation in the context of both your overall practice ratios and, as we mentioned in the previous chapter, your overall staff productivity.

The ideal situation is for the total of your staff expenses and COGS to be 50% or less of your collected gross while your staff productivity ratio is in the range of $125,000 to $175,000 per employee per year.

The undesirable situation is for the total of your staff expenses and COGS to exceed 50% of your collected gross while your staff productivity ratio is below $125,000 per employee per year. That tells me your payroll is too high and your team productivity is too low.

It's also a concern if your staff salaries exceed the practice net income.

Practice net versus owner's net

If you're a solo practice owner, net income is defined as everything that accrues to your personal benefit as an owner. That includes: your salary, profits, retirement plan contributions such as 401K and profit sharing, insurance, and any personal expenses you pay through the practice as legitimate tax deductions.

If you're a solo practice owner, your owner's net equals your practice net. For example:

$1,000,000 gross revenue

- 700,000 expenses

$300,000 = 30% owner's net

If you're a practice owner with the same overhead structure but also have an employed OD, your practice net is still 30%, but your owner's net changes by the amount you pay your associate OD.

$1,000,000 revenue

- 700,000 expenses

300,000 = 30% practice net

- 90,000 employed OD

$210,000 = owner's net

In this case, the owner pays his employed OD $90,000 so his owner's net reduces by that amount.

How Much Should I Pay My Staff?

Therefore, the practice net is 30%, but the owner's net is only $300,000 - $90,000 = $210,000 or 21%.

If you're in a 50/50 partnership with the same overhead structure, your practice net is still 30%, but your personal net changes by the amount you offer each shareholder.

$1,000,000 revenue

-700,000 expenses

$300,000 = 30% practice net

In this case, the two owners split $300,000 equally = $150,000.

$150,000 = 15% net for owner #1

$150,000 = 15% net for owner #2

We point this out so optometrists in larger practices with multiple doctors don't expect their personal net to remain at 30% of total practice revenue. While the absolute amount of dollars you earn should increase as you add associates or partners, your net as a percent of total practice revenues will decline.

How to Measure and Improve Staff Productivity

Chapter highlights:

1. The staff expense category includes everything you spend on your employees including FICA, bonuses, health insurance, retirement programs, travel, training, and uniforms.
2. Staff is your second biggest overhead category, but look at this as an investment, not an expense.
3. The combination of what you spend on your staff and cost of goods should not exceed 50% of your gross collected revenues.

Chapter 6

Keeping Your Salaries in Line

Dear Jerry,

Based on the numbers, my staff salaries seem high at 28% for a $1,000,000 revenue practice. The problem is I have several long-term employees, and I want to pay well so we can provide a high level of service to my patients.

What do you recommend for a situation like mine?

High Roller in Raleigh

Keeping Your Salaries in Line

As we discussed in the previous chapter, a private practice dispensing OD needs to keep the sum of Cost Of Goods and Staff Expenses at or below 50% of total revenues if they want to net 30%. 28% for staff salaries would be high for most practices, but it's perfectly fine if your overhead looks like this:

Collected Gross Income		$1,000,000
COGS	22%	220,000
Staff	28%	280,000
Fixed Overhead	20%	200,000
Total Expenses	70%	700,000
Practice Net	30%	$300,000

Note that 28% for staff expenses works in this case because COGS are only 22% of gross that gives the practice a 'good' ratio of 50% for the sum of staff and

How to Measure and Improve Staff Productivity

COGS. Combined with fixed overhead of 20%, that allows the practice to net 30%.

When are your staff expenses too high?

However, 22% for COGS is lower than average for the majority of practices, so what usually happens when staff expenses exceed 25% of revenues is that you end up netting less than 30% like the example below;

Collected Gross Income		$1,000,000
COGS	30%	300,000
Staff	28%	280,000
Fixed Overhead	20%	200,000
Total Expenses	78%	780,000
Practice Net	22%	$220,000

In this case, the total staff expense is 28% of revenues, or $280,000, while the practice net is 22% or $220,000. In other words, the staff in this practice

Keeping Your Salaries in Line

is making more than the doctor (or doctors), and that is clear sign their overhead ratios are out of line.

Optometrists who find themselves in this situation need to put a long-term emphasis on getting their practice back to normal levels of profitability. That's because a low net income as a percent of your total gross affects not just your take home pay, but your ability to fund your own growth as well as the valuation of your practice.

Three ways staff productivity gets out of line

There are typically three ways the ratio of staff salaries to overall practice revenue can get so out of line:

- Low staff productivity. As we discussed in chapter 3, your practice should produce somewhere between $125,000 to $175,000 per full time employee. That means a solo practice grossing $800,000 will require roughly 5 to 6 employees.

    $800,000 gross ÷ $150,000 = 5.3 employees

Let's assume you have five employees and they make an average of $32,000 per year. That means your total payroll is $160,000 ($32,000 X 5), or 20% of your practice gross.

How to Measure and Improve Staff Productivity

But, what if a different practice had the same pay scale, but only produced $100,000 per employee? That would require eight employees ($800,000 ÷ $100,000).

The payroll in this practice would be $32,000 X 8 employees = $256,000 or 32% of collected gross income.

- Overpaying new hires. Let's say you find yourself short handed and in the interview process with a particularly sharp applicant. When you're feeling desperate for good help, that attractive, well spoken job candidate can look like a savior. So what if they want $45,000 and you had really only planned to pay $40,000? You need somebody now! This phenomenon even has a name, the Halo Effect, and we'll talk about that more in chapter 10.
- Salary creep. The truth is, high staff costs in an optometric office aren't typically caused by low productivity, or a sudden increase due to hiring a big-ticket office manager. In most cases, the problem develops as the salaries of long-term employees 'creep' up over time. I've seen more cases than I can count where long-term employees receiving 5% compounded annual raises attain salary levels that far exceed the market value of their positions.

Keeping Your Salaries in Line

Here's how it happens—let's say you hire a new optician and start him or her at $30,000 per year—then, he performs well, and you give consistently him 5% raises per year. As you can see from the bar graph in Figure 8, his salary will grow from $30,000 to $38,300 in five years, to $48,900 in ten years, and to $79,600 in twenty years.

Salary Creep

Start	5 Years	10 Years	20 Years
$30,000	$38,300	$48,900	$79,600

Fig. 8

A big reason the salary creep problem is so prevalent in well-established practices is because we are dealing with people we like and long-term relationships—not raw statistics consultants like me write about. I have a number of employees with twenty plus years of tenure in my own company, and I know firsthand that balancing cost of living raises with promotions and raises over time is always a challenge.

How to Measure and Improve Staff Productivity

Compassion is admirable and I encourage you to treat your staff well. However, good business sense combined with your ability to match an employee's compensation to the level of contribution they make is required to maintain the overall success and profitability of your practice.

One way to analyze an employee's salary

There are three questions you need to ask yourself when a long-term employee's salary starts to get out of line with what you would pay a new hire for the position:

1. What do other optometrists pay similar employees for this position? See the Prima Staff Salary Survey, or other industry sources for that information.
2. What is the market value for that position in my community?
3. How much is that individual worth to my practice?

In the example below, all their ratios are in line with our suggested benchmarks.

Collected Gross Income		$1,000,000
COGS	28%	280,000
Staff	22%	220,000
Fixed Overhead	20%	200,000

Keeping Your Salaries in Line

Total Expenses	70%	700,000
Practice Net	30%	$300,000

Now, let's say we are doing a salary review of an office manager named Natalie who is currently making $38,000 per year. We compare that to the median salary for office managers in the 2014 Salary Survey conducted by Prima Eye Group that happens to be $40,400. This tells us that Natalie's current pay is $2,400 below the Prima benchmark, and suggests that we have room to increase her base salary depending on some other key factors.

Next, we need to take prevailing salaries for your community into consideration. Wages happen to be higher in Manhattan than they are in Mississippi. An easy way to benchmark that information is by calling a local employment agency. They'll know exactly the prevailing rates for generic office positions such as receptionists and bookkeepers in your area.

Since your local employment agency will likely not have good benchmarks for positions such as frames stylists and optometric assistants, you can look at the optometric surveys and adjust that up or down based on wages in your community that you can compare. For example, if the agency tells you receptionists in your area make an average of $14 an hour and that happens to 5% more than the median wages for receptionists on the Prima Staff Salary Survey, you can adjust the wages up for frame stylists by the same 5%.

Finally, you'll need to make your own judgment call as to how Natalie is performing in your practice relative to her tenure and experience level. If she is a first year employee and you rate her performance as merely average, I would give her no more than a cost of living raise. If she has been with you for several years and doing a good job, then you should consider raising her to near the national average. Likewise, if she has been with you for a long time and is invaluable to the office, then you need to consider paying her in the 80th percentile of the survey range.

Does higher pay lead to better performance?

On the other hand, what if Natalie is performing at what you determine to be an average level but making $55,000 for a position that averages $40,400 on the Prima Staff Salary Survey? And, to make it even worse, your staff costs are 30%, resulting in a practice net of only 25%. This is a classic case of the staff making more than the doctors. And, as I mentioned before, it's a problem for your practice.

At this point, I want you to picture in your mind's eye a guy waving a big red flag. If he looks familiar, that's because it's me! You have exceeded your staff salary budget and must keep your office manager's compensation in line, or your net income will continue to suffer over the long term.

Keeping Your Salaries in Line

Again, lower net affects not just your take home pay, but also your ability to reinvest in your business as you grow and hire an associate—also what your practice will appraise for in a sale or partnership. So, there are lots of good reasons to keep your overhead ratios in line beyond just your own income.

In most cases, practice owners defend their higher than average payrolls by telling me they pay more because they want to provide a high level of service to their patients. I would be all for that if I had some tangible evidence that better than average salaries somehow correlate with superior service levels and higher productivity in optometric offices across the country. But, I don't.

Like many other small business owners, optometrists make the classic mistake of thinking that because they are money motivated, their employees are too. After all, didn't your new receptionist negotiate hard for a higher hourly rate when she was recently hired? And, don't all your employees make it clear they want raises on a regular basis?

No doubt everybody on your payroll wants higher wages. But, that doesn't mean paying them more will directly translate into them working harder and smarter. Here's why:

Everyone has an income threshold

Every worker has a so called personal income threshold. That threshold might be $25,000 a year for your new receptionist, $250,000 for a high producing optometrist and $2,500,000 for the average second baseman in Major League Baseball. Once that threshold is met, simply making more money ceases to be the main motivator. Other factors such as recognition, status, and personal fulfillment become more important than a bigger paycheck.

Let's assume that you are interviewing a sharp young lady for the position of frame stylist, and her personal income threshold is $18 an hour. That is a little bit more than you want to pay, but because she really needs the job, she accepts your offer of $16 per hour. But guess what? If $18 is her felt need, she is going to be a little disappointed with the fact that you out negotiated her, and this could affect her job satisfaction and possibly her performance. She might even keep her eyes open for a better paying position after she comes to work for you. However, you're a smart boss, so you review her after 90 days and decide to bump her to $18 an hour based on good performance. That will be well received, and it will go a long way toward making your new employee feel more content and secure with her job in your office.

But, what if you think she's so good, and you raise her to $20 an hour after ninety days. Will that make her even more happy and productive? The research I've studied suggests that the answer is no.

Keeping Your Salaries in Line

Once you cross the income threshold for someone's base pay, more money does not increase their performance or job satisfaction. If you want to read more on this topic, I highly recommend *Drive: The Surprising Truth About What Motivates Us* by best selling author Daniel Pink.

Of course, everyone's income threshold increases over time based on their progress in the job, and what they see others around them making. So $18 an hour may be great for your frame stylist today, and slightly unsatisfactory to her a year from now. The important point to grasp here is that once the money you give someone for their base pay—the extrinsic motivator—exceeds their current income threshold, then intrinsic motivators such as meaningful work and personal fulfillment become more important influences on extra effort than the pay itself.

Take the average major league second baseman making $2.5 million per year that we cited earlier as an example. There is a story every day in the sports section about a professional ball player holding out for a bigger contract because he feels 'disrespected' by the puny offer of $10 million over four years his team just made. Considering this guy is in his twenties, has no college degree, and his next best career option is making $10 an hour working the graveyard shift at a convenience store, his dissatisfaction is not really about the money. It's all about his expectation of the prestige and recognition relative to where the value of his contract slots him to other players at his position.

Another common example straight out of the sports pages is the player who signs a new multimillion dollar contract only to see his performance on the field fail to live up to his previous press clippings. Once he got the extra money, his effort actually becomes less, not more, than it was before.

Imagine trying to motivate a weak employee who is making $12 an hour by calling her in for a review and giving her a raise her to $24 an hour. Do you really feel her performance will improve dramatically? I don't. In most cases, she's underperforming because: a) you've got her in the wrong position, or b) she's just not that sharp to begin with.

So, no, overpaying your staff will not assure a superior level of team productivity and customer service in your practice.

Now let's take this exercise one step further. What if you raise that weak performer from $12 an hour to $15 and she shows a noticeable improvement in attitude and performance? That tells me you underestimated her personal income threshold and, if that's is the case, I think giving her a raise is smart business. Why? Because high performing employees

Keeping Your Salaries in Line

are what allow you to leverage your personal production.

When staff salaries are 20% of gross collected revenues, you are getting a 5:1 return on your investment. If staff salaries are 25% of revenues, that represents a 4:1 ROI. Anywhere in that range is a good financial return for you.

How much can you afford to pay your staff?

These examples are designed to emphasize the key point of this chapter, and it pays to put some effort into matching the amount you can afford to pay your staff and, at the same time, maximize practice profitability. And, that's where I think most practice owners with high staff salaries get themselves in trouble. They really don't have a good basis for what they should be paying in terms of their own practice overhead, or the local market for each position in their office.

A good place to start is by reviewing your practice overhead. Is the sum of your staff expenses cost of goods 50% or more of your gross collected revenues?

Next, which is higher, the doctors' net or total staff expenses?

How to Measure and Improve Staff Productivity

Then look at hard data like the staff salary survey from Prima that tells you what other private practice optometrists are paying their team members.

Finally, compare that data with the salary levels provided by employment agencies in your area. Once you are on solid ground with what you should be paying, job applicants can decide for themselves if your offer meets their income threshold.

7 ways to keep staff salaries in line

It's no surprise that the optometrists we work with who are most concerned about salary creep are the ones who are dealing with it. You likely didn't get yourself in this situation overnight, and there is no quick fix to get out of it. But, any practice owner can correct the problem and get ratios under control over time. It just requires holding the line on big raises, and possibly turning over some staff.

The best solution to the problem of salary creep is, of course, not to get in that position in the first place! Here are seven simple guidelines to help you keep your staff tenure and compensation in balance:

1. As an employer, you pay people for two things: how well they do their jobs, and how they impact practice revenues. It's your job to decide how each member of your team rates on those criteria.
2. Every position has a market value—stay current with the prevailing wages in your area

Keeping Your Salaries in Line

and use hard data such as the Staff Salary Survey from Prima Eye Group to benchmark your payroll. Paying above market value may make it easier to hire and retain someone, but it won't assure superior performance.

3. Avoid awarding raises simply based on length of service. Cost of living increases are generally in the range of 2% to 3% per year. Depending on someone's base pay relative to national norms, a 4% to 5% raise should require an employee to master new skills and improve measurably at their current tasks.
4. When an employee's performance plateaus, so should their compensation. It only took you four years to get through optometry school. Even your best employees' skill level will top out at three-to-five years if they stay in the same position. Make sure you give them every possible opportunity to grow in the job.
5. Be a boss, not a friend. Your employees work in your office for their own reasons. Don't get so tied up in their personal lives that you feel an obligation to pay them a certain amount.
6. Don't exaggerate any one staff member's importance to the success of your practice. Overdependence on a key employee puts you in position of weakness and it's never a good

thing for your practice. This goes beyond someone's pay—what happens if they quit, move, or die?
7. Don't expect to make all your people, even the good ones, lifetime employees. Sometimes it's in the best interest of both your practice and the person for a long-term employee to move on.

In closing, compensation issues are one of the most difficult management items a practice owner has to deal with. My goal in this chapter was to give you a thought process and methodology you can use to get a handle on where your staff salaries should be.

Chapter highlights:

1. Most optometrists who spend more than 50% of their gross on the sum of cost of goods and staff, net less than 30%.
2. Staff salaries tend to creep up over time because the employee's skill level doesn't grow at the same rate as their pay increases.
3. Paying above market value may make it easier to hire and retain someone, but it won't assure superior performance.

Chapter 7

Do Staff Bonuses Really Work?

Dear Jerry,

We've tried several different bonus programs for our staff over the years with varying degrees of success. Do you think bonuses are really necessary? And, if so, can you recommend a good plan to put in place?

Happy in Hattiesburg

Do Staff Bonuses Really Work?

At this point, let's say your overhead ratios look good and your base salaries are in line with the national norms for each position in your practice. Does it make sense to institute a bonus program that gives your staff extra pay for extra performance?

Optometrists are all over the map when it comes to what type of bonus plan to use, if any. According to a survey conducted by the Management & Business Academy, sixty percent of private practice ODs give some sort of financial bonus to their staff every year. The average bonus was reported at 4% of base salary. Example: $35,000 x 4% = $1,400.

While no details were provided on what the bonuses were based on, or when they were given, 29% of the responding ODs reported that their bonus programs were <u>extremely</u> effective while 62% said their bonus programs were <u>very</u> effective.

It sounds good, but I don't buy it.

Why your bonus plan doesn't work

Oh, sure, I think every staff member loves getting a bonus. So, if the definition of 'effective' is pleasing your staff, I'll go along. But, if the definition of 'effective' is improving team productivity and getting better financial results for your practice, most of the staff bonus programs I see are not that well designed.

Which goes back to the original questions—do bonuses really work, and are they necessary to have a happy and productive team?

Based on my experience, yes, a well-constructed staff bonus program can help improve productivity and increase profits. But, no—I do not think bonus programs are necessary to have a successful practice, nor are they a panacea for motivating an underperforming team.

The same concepts we discussed about income thresholds in the previous chapter apply to bonuses. Some people are very money motivated, and others not so much. You, no doubt, have both kinds in your office. And, you likely get frustrated when some of your employees don't work harder or push certain products to achieve the financial incentives you created for them.

We've all hired notable exceptions, but the kind of person who accepts a job in your office for $10 - $15 - $20 an hour is generally not that money motivated beyond their income threshold. If they were, they wouldn't come to work for you in the first place. They would get a commission based sales job with Mary Kay™ or at a store in the mall where their pay links directly to some sales goal. However, by the process of self-selection, the people you hire don't want to do that, they prefer to make a fixed hourly rate; and, the fact that they can help others by serving patients in a doctor's office is important to them.

So, it's vital to keep in mind that the attitude most of your hourly staff has about money—and, how to make it—is significantly different from someone like you who owns a small business or optometric practice and works for themselves.

In the previous chapter, we said the income threshold might be $25,000 a year for your new receptionist, $250,000 for a high-producing optometrist in his own practice, and $2,500,000 for the average second baseman in Major League Baseball. Of course, salary expectations will increase over time, but once someone's base pay exceeds their current income threshold, intrinsic factors such as the ability to control their own work, belonging to a team, and helping others then becomes more important motivators of extra effort than the pay itself.

Why do bonuses work?

However, let's not throw the baby out with the bath water. Bonus programs can and do work for three important reasons: one, extrinsic motivators like money may not be a person's main driver, but a little part of everybody will respond to a 'you do this and I'll give you that' financial carrot. Just not to the degree you may want them to.

Two, humans are goal seeking organisms—it's just the way we're built. And, an inherent part of every good bonus system is a measurable objective. The example would be giving your dispensing optician a $10 bonus for every $300 frame they sell. Helping patients pick out a $300 frame then becomes the goal, not making $10. The extra money is great, but for most of your team, it's the clearly stated objective—you want to sell $300 frames—that influences behavior and gets results.

Three, success leads to personal recognition by the boss and status in the office. Your employees *want* money, they *crave* recognition and status. Every time they make a certain number of appointments or sell the right frame, they've accomplished something and won your approval in the process. For these people, the extra money that goes with the bonus is the icing, but the good feeling that goes with achieving their goal as well as the positive feedback they get from pleasing you is the cake itself.

The type of bonus affects your culture

It's also important to keep in mind that your reward system will directly affect the culture of your office. The more you incentivize your team with money for specific activities such as selling $300 frames or expensive lenses, the more likely you are to instill a sales mentality in your office. And, for sure, you are going to get a lot of encouragement from your frame and lab reps to use those type of incentives; they are, after all, trained sales people and their main interest is moving product.

On the other hand, motivational tools such as clearly defined goals, praise, and recognition help you build an attitude of service. I'm not presenting this as a good or bad, right or wrong way to do things. I've seen both approaches employed with a high degree of success in optometric practices. But, it is important to think about the kind of culture you want to nurture in your practice.

4 ways to improve your bonus program

Odds are, you are in the 60% that already has some type of staff bonus program in your practice. If so, keep doing what works for you. Likewise, if you don't have a bonus program now, this is not an attempt to convince you to implement one. However, if you want to tweak the program you have, or maybe see how your team will respond to bonuses, I have four suggestions on how to make a bonus program more effective and get your staff aligned with your financial objectives in the process.

1 - Reward results, not activities.

It's very common for ODs to bonus their staff on revenue generating events such as how many appointments they make, or how many $300 frames,

AR coatings, or second pairs they sell. I am not a fan of this approach because, these are merely activities, and what I am interested in is results. Yes, they are important activities, but some practices sell a lot of high-end frames and lenses and still make below average profits.

Bottom line, there is a lot more that goes into building a profitable, high volume practice, such as delivering a superior patient experience, than how many expensive glasses you sell. So, why not create your staff bonus program around the financial results you want and can easily measure? They are:

1. Higher practice revenues
2. Higher gross profits
3. Higher net profits

2 - *Bonus the team, not the individual!*

The best way I know of to motivate and unify a team is to create team goals and a shared reward system. For that reason, I don't like the idea of a bonus system that rewards your opticians, but not your receptionists, assistants, and bookkeepers. A system that recognizes only a select few has the potential to foster jealously and it certainly makes it harder to develop a sense of teamwork among your whole staff. The exception might be if you have a mega office with dozens of employees and different departments. But if you have less than ten employees, offering a performance bonus to some and not to others can create problems.

Do Staff Bonuses Really Work?

Sometimes practice owners tell me they give one employee a bonus because they do more than others. I don't expect you to pay everybody the same, but if you feel someone is more valuable to your practice, simply increase their base salary.

3 - *The goal is more important than the reward!*

As we have already said, for many people a clearly stated objective will often do more to influence behavior and get results than a monetary bonus. Case in point—Dr. Neil Gailmard built one of the highest producing professional practices in the country with virtually no reliance on staff bonus programs. Employees at the Gailmard Eye Center, however, do have clearly defined outcome goals.

4 - *Keep your bonus criteria clear and simple!*

Optometrists, by and large, are very intelligent and if smart people like anything, they love complexity. This, in fact, is a very common problem in all businesses—clever people have a tendency to make things more complicated than they need to be. I advise you to keep your staff bonus program as simple as possible.

True story—I recently consulted with the owner of a $1 million practice with a rather complex staff bonus program. I do this stuff every day, and it was frankly difficult for me to follow the ifs, ands, and buts of the program as she talked me through it.

How to Measure and Improve Staff Productivity

Although her practice was doing well and she assured me her staff loved the bonus system, I was skeptical. My suspicions were confirmed when I talked to a staff member in private and she told me, yes, they liked the bonus program. They just couldn't explain how it worked or what they got their bonus check for. Which tells me the doctor had not done a good job of tying the money she spends on bonuses to clearly defined outcome goals.

A simple incentive program

To illustrate how an easy to understand bonus program can work, let's create a fictional practice owner called Dr. Biggers, and build a sample plan using my four principles of results, teamwork, clear goals, and simplicity.

We'll assume Dr. Biggers's practice grossed $944,000 last year, and his COGS were 31%. He's had a sales based bonus system in place for his opticians, and has now decided he wants to replace that with team goals as well as a shared reward for his entire staff based on two of our three criteria:

- Higher practice revenues
- Cost of Goods

I've left net profit out on purpose because I know most ODs don't want to share that information with their employees, and I understand that. So, we substitute Cost of Goods, which is the inverse of

Do Staff Bonuses Really Work?

gross profits, for the employee goals. This simplifies the program even more, and gives us the same effect.

Another reason to leave net profits out of your staff goal is that you always want to bonus people on things they control, and your staff has little say in how much you spend on rent, marketing, equipment, and staff salaries. But, your staff is very involved in managing the frame and lens inventory in your practice which is why I like to use Cost of Goods as the expense component of my staff bonus program.

There are two ways Dr. Biggers can decide on what his goals for gross revenues and cost of goods should be. He can do the math all by himself and just present his numbers to the staff.

Or, he can discuss his criteria with his office manager and other key team members to let them give input about what the goals should be. I like this approach for two reasons: one, getting your staff to buy in on the front end assures a higher level of commitment to the process. Two, doctors frequently find their staff to be more aggressive and optimistic about practice growth than expected. You can always negotiate the goals with your staff if you feel they are unrealistically high or low.

Let's say Dr. Biggers meets with his key staff members and, after much discussion, they decide to shoot for a six percent increase in revenues. That

How to Measure and Improve Staff Productivity

makes his revenue goal 1.06 X $944,000 = $1,000,000 for the year.

Set your goals on a quarterly basis

The next step for Dr. Biggers is to break the revenues for the previous year into increments of three months each—accountants call this quarters—so he can apply a six percent increase and set his revenue goal for next year. I advise you to break your revenue goals into quarters because your staff will lose patience with annual goals, and the number of working days per month varies from year to year making it hard to compare apples to apples from each month of one year to the next. Example:

Q1 - 6% increase = $260,000 revenue
Q2 - 6% increase = $240,000 revenue
Q3 - 6% increase = $270,000 revenue
Q4 - 6% increase = $230,000 revenue

Total = $1,000,000 for the year

These numbers then become the 'production goals' that tell your team how much you have to bring in each quarter to hit the revenue component of your staff bonus program.

But, revenue is only half the story of any profit and loss statement. That's why we also put in a criteria for Cost of Goods. I feel very strongly about including an expense control component to your

Do Staff Bonuses Really Work?

bonus program, especially for practices that net less than 30%.

There is no magic formula for how much you should reduce your COGS number. If yours is 30% or above, I would try to reduce it a percent or two. So, after meeting, Dr. Biggers, his staff decides their COGS goal will be 31 – 1 = 30%.

The intention is to grow revenues by six percent, and decrease expenses by one percent knowing that when these two things happen, his gross profits will increase by $49,000 over the year.

$1,000,000 - 30% COGS = $700,000
$ 944,000 - 31% COGS = $651,000
$ 700,000 - $651,000 = $ 49,000

So, now we have two result oriented goals, a six percent increase in gross collected revenues for each quarter along with gross profits of 70% which we express to the staff as COGS expense of no more than 30%.

Q1 - $260,000 revenue with 30% COGS
Q2 - $240,000 revenue with 30% COGS
Q3 - $270,000 revenue with 30% COGS
Q4 - $230,000 revenue with 30% COGS

Total = $1,000,000 for the year

How to Measure and Improve Staff Productivity

At this point, Dr. Biggers and his staff have set financial goals for the year. I cannot emphasize enough what a powerful exercise this discussion is for the success of his practice. If you haven't done this yourself this year, please stop and do it now!

If you're doing this for the first time, I highly recommend that you let your key employees, if not your entire staff, know what your expectations are for practice revenue and gross profits in the form of Cost of Goods expense. Why? Something magic happens when the leader of any organization presents a shared goal to a team of people. It sounds simple, but humans are goal-seeking organisms and your practice goals are what get your team—and, you—working toward a common purpose. Don't skip this step because it really works.

How much to bonus?

Now, what about the bonus side of the equation? How can we translate our desired financial results into a bonus plan that rewards our team when we achieve a shared financial goal?

If you're in the forty percent of practice owners that don't give financial bonuses to your team and your practice is achieving the results you want, I don't recommend that you suddenly tack a big financial reward onto to your planning process.

I do strongly suggest that you celebrate your successes. Maybe it's something simple like ordering pizza for the staff or taking everybody to lunch and

Do Staff Bonuses Really Work?

make a big deal of it when you meet your quarterly goals. Then do a nice dinner with spouses when you make your annual goal. Whatever you do, make a point to recognize your accomplishments, and praise your staff whenever your practice has a good month or good year. That type of recognition and praise goes a long way toward keeping your staff motivated.

If you're in the sixty percent that are already giving financial bonuses and you want to continue that tradition, I urge you to tie the bonus to some number that directly correlates to your goals. What I generally suggest for a revenue-based program like Dr. Biggers's is to bonus your staff one percent of revenues each quarter you hit both goals.

In other words, as you present your practice goals, tell your team that each quarter you hit your targets for gross collected revenue AND cost of goods, they will split one percent of revenues.

Q1 - $260,000 revenue with 30% COGS
Q2 - $240,000 revenue with 30% COGS
Q3 - $270,000 revenue with 30% COGS
Q4 - $230,000 revenue with 30% COGS

Total = $1,000,000 for the year

In Dr. Biggers's case, reaching their first quarter goal would create a bonus pool of $2,600.

How to Measure and Improve Staff Productivity

$260,000 X 1% = $2,600

Let's say he had eight employees, six full time and two who work half time each for a total of seven full time equivalent (FTE) employees. The six full timers would each get a full share, and the two part timers would each get a half share for a total of seven full shares.

Therefore, the bonus calculation for this quarter would be $2,600 ÷ 7 FTEs = $371.

In this case, each full time employee would get a full share of $371, and the two part timers would get a fractional share of $185.50 ($371 ÷ 2).

You would then repeat the process each quarter. If you hit your revenue goal, but not your COGS, I suggest giving your team 50% of the bonus. But, if you don't hit your revenue goal, there is no reward that quarter.

However, if you miss your revenue goal one quarter, but achieve both goals for the year, I suggest giving the full bonus at year end minus whatever you already paid.

$371 isn't a huge bonus, but it is going to get the attention of a person making $15 to $20 an hour. As I have already made the case for many people, it's the clearly stated objective that influences behavior and gets results, not the monetary bonus. A program like this also assumes you are paying all of your staff at or near their personal income threshold. None of your

Do Staff Bonuses Really Work?

employees should be looking at this bonus as guaranteed or part of their base salary.

Stick to it

One of the most frequent complaints I hear about bonus plans from practice owners is—it doesn't mean anything anymore, and my staff has come to expect it. When that's the case, it's probably your fault because: a) the results weren't tied directly to practice growth, b) the criteria wasn't clear, or c) you caved and paid up whether your practice achieved the goal or not.

For that reason, it's very important to tell your staff on the front end, the numbers are the numbers. You get paid a fixed salary for your daily efforts and the bonus is extra if we achieve our goals. I don't want to hear how hard you worked, how many no shows we had, or how bad the weather was. The revenues we generate fund the bonus pool, and we either make it or we don't. As Yoda famously said in *Star Wars*—"Do, or do not. There is no try."

Should you bonus your team?

My example of the 1% quarterly bonus is only one way to do it. Opinions vary widely on what constitutes a good bonus program and how effective they really are. Monetary bonuses definitely work for some people. But they aren't absolutely necessary to get good results out of your staff. Clearly defined outcome goals are, however, very important for practice owners who want to get the best of their team.

It's also important to keep in mind that whatever money you invest in your staff in the form of a bonus program will fall under the staff salaries category and will add to your overall staff expense.

Chapter highlights:

1. Well-constructed bonus programs can work, but you don't need to pay bonuses to have a highly successful practice.
2. A good bonus program should focus on results leading to an increase in practice revenues and profits, not merely activities.
3. Your bonus program should be simple to explain, and easy to understand with a minimum of complexity.

Chapter 8

Give Your Team a Sense of Purpose

Dear Jerry,

My office manager recently told me she does not approve of some fee increases I made. She actually accused me of being more concerned with how much money we make than providing good care to our patients. I take patient care and customer service very seriously, and I'm shocked she would say something like that. I need some suggestions, and a pep talk!

Worried in Washington

Give Your Team A Sense of Purpose

It is definitely a concern when a team member questions your commitment to patient care, especially when it comes from your office manager, the person you expect to set an example for everyone else in the practice.

This was a real case and when I looked at Dr. Washington's overhead, I saw that her practice net was only 24%, while her staff salaries were 30%. In other words, her staff was making more than she was, and her overhead ratios were out of line. All to say, the office manager's concern that the doctor is profiteering at the expense of patients is greatly misplaced.

Let's revisit what you, as the owner of an optometric practice, really want from your team:

- High level of service to patients
- Good return on investment
- Peace and harmony

It's fair to say that Dr. Washington and her team are out of alignment on all three: one, the office manager is accusing the doctor of being more concerned with money than serving patients. Two, because of her low net, the doctor is getting a below average return on investment. Three, they certainly are not at peace with each other.

How to Measure and Improve Staff Productivity

The big question is how does the doctor get the office manager and the rest of her team in alignment with her practice goals?

I recently heard Shahid Khan, the owner of the Jacksonville Jaguars football team, speak about entrepreneurship. Here's a guy who immigrated to the United States from Pakistan at age 16 and got his start washing dishes at the YMCA for $1.20 an hour. He is now a billionaire, an NFL owner, and the CEO of Flex-N-Gate, an auto parts manufacturer with 17,000 employees in 13 countries. Mr. Khan said he looks for two things in the people he hires—the desire to make a difference in the lives of others, and the ability to help his businesses make money. I submit that you want the same attitudes in the employees in your practice.

You can use the concepts we discussed in Chapter 7 to create financial objectives around revenues and cost control for your team. We'll devote this chapter to talking about three specific steps you can take to build a culture of customer service, and make it crystal clear to your team that you are committed to making a difference in the lives of the patients you serve.

1 - Define the purpose of your practice

In his excellent book, *Drive: The Surprising Truth About What Motivates Us,* best-selling author Daniel Pink makes the case that the secret to high

Give Your Team a Sense of Purpose

performance and satisfaction at work, school, and home is the deeply human need to direct our own lives, learn and create new things, do better by ourselves, and to help others. I believe that, and I try to apply that concept when leading my own team.

A problem that Dr. Washington shares with many other practice owners is that she hasn't clearly and formally articulated the purpose of her practice. Yes, we all assume that you are there to provide excellent eyecare to all your patients and, in the process, make enough profits to afford good staff salaries, a nice office, and modern equipment. But, when those goals are stated in a rather general way, or, in many cases, not stated at all, they tend to get lost while you're team is dealing with dozens of demanding people over the course of a busy day.

Many highly successful doctors have such a clear picture in their own head of how they want things to be, they find it easy to lead by example and communicate a well-defined vision of success to their staff without putting anything in writing. But, what if you're a little fuzzy yourself about the true purpose of your practice, and if you're sure about anything, it's that your team is not on the same page with you?

If you suspect that you're not fully in sync with your staff on objectives for customer service and overall practice performance, it's a good idea to

How to Measure and Improve Staff Productivity

spend some time with your team creating a Purpose Statement. This is actually a simpler version of what many companies call a Mission Statement. Shown is a copy of the Purpose Statement that Apple gives to all new employees.

> **Apple's™ Purpose Statement**
>
> There's work and there's your life's work.
>
> The kind of work that has your fingerprints all over it. The kind of work that you'd never compromise on. That you'd sacrifice a weekend for.
>
> You can do that kind of work at Apple. People don't come here to play it safe. They come here to swim in the deep end.
>
> They want their work to add up to something. Something big. Something that couldn't happen anywhere else.
>
> Welcome to Apple.

Fig. 9

The obvious goal of Apple's purpose statement is to pre-sell—some would say indoctrinate—new employees with the idea that you are being asked to give the level of commitment that Steve Jobs was famous for demanding. This kind of straight talking purpose statement appeals to people who come to work at Apple because they want to make a difference in the world. In this case, serving mankind through technology. But, this type of formalized statement can also work very well for health care providers. Mayo Clinic publishes the following Mission, Vision, and Value Statements on their website.

Give Your Team a Sense of Purpose

> **Mayo Clinic™**
> **Mission, Vision, Value Statement**
>
> **Mission** — to inspire hope, and contribute to health and well-being by providing the best care to every patient through integrated clinical practice, education, and research.
>
> **Vision** — Mayo Clinic will provide an unparalleled experience as the most trusted partner for health care.
>
> **Value** — the needs of the patient come first.

Fig. 10

So, one very tangible step you can take to build a strong culture of service in your practice is to follow the example of these two world-class organizations and craft your own Purpose Statement. Depending on the size of your team, you can meet with all or some of your staff to create your own version. It won't be etched in stone, so don't make this a bigger project than it needs to be, or try to word it perfectly. Example:

> **The Family Eye Center – Sample**
>
> Our purpose at the Family Eye Center is to provide the best possible eyecare and the highest quality eyewear services to the patients who entrust their visual welfare to us on a daily basis.
>
> We provide those services in a friendly and pleasant manner that makes our patients feel both valued as individuals and appreciated for the business they give us.

Fig. 11

How to Measure and Improve Staff Productivity

The goal is to put something on paper that you can point to every time you need to remind your employees of why you all come to work every day. Use my example if you need somewhere to start.

2 - Use stories to build a strong culture

The second important step toward building a strong culture in your practice is to tell stories about the things that make your practice special in the eyes of patients. Here is one of my favorites from the retail industry: the Discount Rack of Nordstrom's Department Store took over the space formerly occupied by a tire shop in Fairbanks, AK, and a new employee was assigned to work the returns desk. A customer comes in, lays two snow tires on the counter and asks for a refund. The clerk, fresh out of training and well versed in the importance of providing high level customer service the Nordstrom way, sees a price tag for $145 on the tires and gives the man a full refund without further questions. Never mind that Nordstrom sells high-end clothing and fashion accessories, but not snow tires!

Is this really true? I don't know, but even if it's not, this urban legend has been around long enough to speak volumes about the Nordstrom brand and their reputation for outstanding customer service.

My favorite optometric version of a great customer recovery story was told at a Prima Eye

Give Your Team a Sense of Purpose

Group meeting by my friend, Dr. Howard Day, who owns a practice with his wife, Dr. Sharon Day, in Gardendale, AL. It seems that one of his patients, a young woman of limited means, was wearing – 9.00 diopter OU in frames that were about a year old. She came in for a routine adjustment and as the optician was putting the glasses back on her face, the highly myopic patient noticed a small hairline scratch in lower nasal corner of the right lens. Visibly alarmed, she blurted, "You scratched my glasses!" at the optician. "Yes, I did notice that scratch, but it was already there," he calmly responded. The young woman was sure he had just scratched the lens while cleaning them, and became visibly upset.

The optician remained cool while they discussed her concerns, and he finally asked what the patient wanted him to do. "Fix it" was her only request, so he told her to give him a few days, and he would have a new pair of glasses ready for her.

The Nordstrom legend may not be true, but Dr. Day's story is and it's a great example of a reputation-building story for his optometric practice. You see, Howard's office has a 'patient recovery program' that empowers every member of his staff to spend up to $200 to fix patient complaints and customer service problems on the spot—without getting his approval.

How to Measure and Improve Staff Productivity

Many ODs tell me they wouldn't do this because they are afraid their staff will give away the store, but I think it is a great policy to consider for your office. It's easy enough to set limits and monitor the frequency of use if you are concerned about the expense. I tell ODs to budget 1% of annual revenues for their customer recovery program, and look at it as a low cost marketing program to generate terrific word of mouth advertising. Nobody has ever reported spending that much to me.

Don't have any great stories of your own? Do you like Nordstrom's? Then make one up, or embellish your own urban legend of service if the perfect example didn't really happen in your office. For example, the time Mary drove to the lab in a driving rain to pick up glasses for a patient in desperate need. Or, when Larry, your dispensing optician, agreed to remake a brand new pair of expensive progressive lenses because Aunt Sally changed her mind and decided she didn't like the frame she picked out. Or, the time you made a potentially sight saving diagnosis in a young child during a routine ophthalmoscopy.

It's memorable and effective when you give your staff specific examples of the level of service you expect them to provide in your office. Your team can relate to stories and all you need is one or two good ones you can tell over and over when customer service lapses do occur.

Give Your Team a Sense of Purpose

3 - You have to walk the talk

Here's the third and most important step toward building a culture of customer service in your practice—your daily actions have to serve as an everyday example for your staff. In other words, having a Purpose Statement and inspiring stories of legendary service that occurred in your practice are great, but long term, your staff will not treat patients with more care and attention than you.

What you say and what you do in front of patients, as well as behind their backs is the template your employees will use for their own behavior. Make it a good one.

Chapter highlights:

1. Create a Purpose Statement to get your staff focused on providing a high level of service to your patients.
2. Use stories to reinforce the culture of service you want to maintain in your practice.
3. The practice owner must lead by example.

Chapter 9

Team Meetings

Dear Jerry,

I have a $900,000 practice with seven employees, and we are so busy it's hard to find time for staff meetings. Do you think they are really that important for a successful practice like mine?

Dr. Meeter in Michigan

Team Meetings

In my opinion, regular team meetings are an integral part of the staff management process, especially for a growing practice with more than one or two employees. Staff meetings are the best platform I know of for communicating with your employees, and reinforcing the things you want done in your practice.

A few years after opening, I had five employees and made the classic mistake of calling meetings only when problems or conflicts developed to the point that we had to convene to put out fires. My way of giving feedback at that time was management by wandering around. If someone needed a little training, or if I saw them doing something wrong, I just told them on the spot. But, it was all ad lib and there was no formality or consistency to my process.

Over time, a little personality conflict developed between two women in my office, so I decided to call a staff meeting to discuss their misunderstanding, as well as how it was affecting my other employees. While the session started out with these two ladies angry at each other, a mob mentality soon took over and the whole staff decided to gang up and take their frustrations out on me. I realized then and there that I had let some known problems build up in my busy practice, and morale wasn't that great. The fact is we were long overdue to work on some personnel important issues, and that was the crisis I needed to start having staff meetings on a weekly basis. My advice is not to let it get that far in your office.

How often should you meet?

Even if you have a small practices with only two or three employees, I think you need to meet with every staff member at least once a week. That may sound like a lot, but it's really not for practice owners who consider themselves customer service oriented and want to stay on top of things.

The need to meet personally with every staff member every week might change once you get to ten or more employees in the same office. In that case, you can delegate some of the meetings to a full time office manager. But, for the typical practice with two to nine non-OD staff members, once a week seems about right to me.

By 'meeting' I don't mean lock the front door, turn off the phones, and hunker down for an hour or two. Some practice owners prefer to do it that way, particularly for training sessions, and I have no problem if it works for you. I've just found that it's easy to put off longer meetings when seemingly more urgent matters come up.

Here's the way we did it—once I added my office manager, I had six non-OD staff in my practice. The staff arrived for work at 8:30 AM and we started seeing patients at 9 AM. I would meet for fifteen to thirty minutes with two employees first thing in the

Team Meetings

morning while the others answered the phones and handled the front desk. We did that on a rotating basis every Monday, Wednesday, and Friday which allowed me to cover the whole staff over the course of a week.

Of course, we couldn't always cover everything in those short meetings, so we would have a longer meeting with the whole staff about once a month. That format worked quite well for years in my practice.

What do you talk about?

I've had doctors tell me, *I'm not opposed to meeting with my staff, I just don't know what we would talk about.* There should never be a shortage things to talk about in a busy practice. Sometimes the topics of discussion will be the same for everybody, such as, when we were going to close the office for holidays.

But often, I had different things to discuss based on whether I was meeting with the front desk staff, optical staff, or contact lens staff. Plus, I would not hesitate to meet with someone individually when they needed 'extra coaching' or maybe a little course correction on things they needed to do better.

How to Measure and Improve Staff Productivity

One of my tricks was to keep a little black book in my pocket so I could make notes as different issues came up during the day of things I wanted to discuss

Practice Manager's Weekly Report

For Week: _____ Date: ___ / ___ / ___

Comprehensive exam slots
Comprehensive exams performed
Pairs of new lenses sold
New frames sold
Second pairs sold
Rx walkouts
Capture rate
Contact lens fits

Customer service lapses:

Resolution:

Customer service success stories:

Action steps for next week:

Person responsible:

© 2014 Prima Eye Group

Fig. 12

in the weekly staff meetings. It might be simple things like I wasn't happy with the way our

Team Meetings

receptionist handled a patient on the phone, or how my optician could better present high-end frames to fashion-conscious patients. I'd make my list, and then cover those things in our weekly meetings.

More recently, we've developed something called the Practice Manager's Weekly Report. This is a simple worksheet we use to track key result areas for members of Prima Eye Group. The beauty of this form is that it captures all the production data you need to have for a meaningful discussion in your weekly staff meetings.

I use a form like this when consulting with ODs in Prima because I really believe that measurement is the beginning point for positive change. If you want to improve an area of your practice, start tracking it. If you measure things on a consistent basis patterns will begin to emerge. Once you see a pattern, good or bad, you and your staff will be able to figure out ways to improve on it.

In One Ear, Out the Other

OK, I've made the case that it's great to meet with your staff at least once a week to discuss general housekeeping items, as well as things that need to be done to facilitate the growth of the practice. But, have you ever had the experience of meeting with someone to tell how, when, or where to do something only to have the instructions

How to Measure and Improve Staff Productivity

misunderstood or totally ignored? Of course! We all have. When verbal instructions break down, there are generally three reasons:

1. You know exactly what you want to happen, but your instructions were not clear.

2. The listener was in a passive mode. They were not actively ignoring you. They may have been distracted, or just not engaged in what you had to say.

3. Your instructions were clear, and the listener was engaged. But, they didn't understand, and they weren't assertive enough to ask for clarity.

Use the Mirror Technique to Be Heard

In any case, there is a better way to make sure you are heard called the 'mirror technique.' I actually learned how to do this in a marriage enrichment class with my wife, and am happy to report that she has used it on me with great success over the years. Here is an example of how it works:

Doctor: *Susie, I noticed we are having a lot of no shows lately. I just want to remind you that an important part of your job is to confirm each appointment at least 24 hours in advance. Any questions?*
Susie: *No, I understand.*

Team Meetings

Doctor: *Can you mirror that back to me please? I just want to make sure you understand what I'm asking.*

Susie: *What I heard you say was that it would be a good idea to confirm most of our appointments at least one day in advance. Have I got that right?*

Side note: You need to explain the mirror technique to your staff in advance and teach them to use the phrases, "What I heard you say was . . ." and, "Have I got that right?"

Doctor: *No. I did not say it would be a good idea. What I said was that as part of your job, you must absolutely, positively, confirm every appointment at least 24 hours in advance. I expect you to tell me if there is any reason you cannot do that. Can you mirror that back to me, please?*

Susie: *What I heard you say was that I absolutely, positively, need to confirm every appointment on the books at least 24 hours in advance. And, if for some reason I cannot do that, I need to let you know. Have I got that right?*

Doctor: *Thanks, Susie. You have it!*

    The beauty of the mirror technique is that it forces the other party to stop, think, and engage in

How to Measure and Improve Staff Productivity

the listening process. And, then, it gives the speaker an opportunity to clarify his or her message.

This is also a wonderful technique to use with your employees when they are voicing a complaint or concern. For example:

Brittany: *Dr. Meeter, I've been here a year as a receptionist and I would like to be considered for training as an optometric technician.*

You: *OK, I'm glad to know you're interested. What I heard you say was that you would like to be trained as an optometric technician. Have I got that right?*

Brittany: *Yes, Sir—that would be great.*

This is a simple dialog technique that you can use to make your staff members feel heard. Acknowledge them by repeating what they asked you for, and it's much better than just saying OK, or I'll think about it.

Are you guilty of managing by text?

I got a question recently from a practice owner who said that he had texted a salary proposal to his receptionist and she texted back, "Not happy, I think I am worth more than that to your practice."

I am a big user of technology, but I have to admit that I cringed more than a little over the idea that a practice owner would text a salary proposal to a staff member who is sitting less than 50 feet away.

Team Meetings

The implication is the doctor is too timid to handle salary discussions on a face-to-face basis. If I think that, your employee no doubt senses it and this can work against you in salary negotiations.

I completely understand the human side of this situation because I've had the same problem with a few strong-willed employees who still come to mind. But, it's my opinion that trying to manage your staff by text and email is almost never as good as the old-fashioned face-to-face way.

In the cases where you do avoid confrontation by using texts or email to convey an awkward point, you often create an 'elephant in the room' scenario where you both know there's an unresolved issue, but neither you nor the employee wants to talk about it. I've been there, too, and that type of baggage has a way of adversely affecting employee morale in the entire office.

It's also very easy to come across as blunt or brusque, as well as your being totally misunderstood when you write something in an email or text. Does the reply, 'Not happy' mean the employee would like more, but they'll take it? Or, does it mean, "I have to have more, or I quit?" Those things aren't clear in a short burst e-message.

If you want the best out of your staff, the thing to keep in mind is that you manage processes, but

How to Measure and Improve Staff Productivity

you lead people. There is no better way to establish yourself as the leader of your practice than by communicating face to face on a regular basis with all your staff members. It's not always comfortable, but it's like doing eye examinations—the more you do it, the better results you get. And, the more your employees will respect and respond to you.

Chapter highlights:

1. Weekly staff meetings are an important platform for communicating with your employees and reinforcing the things you want done in your practice.

2. Take notes during the day to remind yourself of things you want to discuss in your weekly meetings.

3. Use the Mirror Technique to get your point across and to make your staff feel heard.

Chapter 10

Holding Your Employees Accountable

Dear Jerry,

I have a problem in that my employees know what to do, but they don't always do it. I call them on it, but sometimes they just don't take me seriously. How can I be a better boss and get my staff to do what I want them to?

The Donald in New York

How to Measure and Improve Staff Productivity

Some ODs are like Rodney Dangerfield—they get no respect in their own office. I can't tell you how many times I've heard comments such as, "Linda just won't do what I ask her to" or, "I would like to try that new practice building idea, but my staff just won't go for it." Early in my career, I was sitting in on one of those spirited group conversations optometrists always seem to have around the bar at state association meetings. We were talking about managing staff and everybody agreed that it was downright difficult to get our employees to do what we wanted them to on a consistent basis. One successful OD told us that he looked every new hire directly in the eye and said, "Are going to do what I tell you to?" His methodology struck me as blunt, but that's about as succinctly as you can put it.

As I said earlier, the first limiting factor to practice growth is an OD's ability to manage a growing staff of employees and getting them to execute your plan. It's where the rubber meets the road. The difference between providing your patients with a mediocre level of service versus a world-class experience in your office is directly related to how well your staff not just listens, but actually does what you want them to.

So, how do you make that happen? Assuming they know what to do and how to do it, your staff is

Holding Your Employees Accountable

going to comply with your wishes for one of three reasons:

1. Your best employees are probably the ones who are compliant by nature and want to do the right thing simply because you ask them to. Why can't they all be that way?
2. Many successful ODs are able to demand staff compliance through the sheer force of their personality. These doctors don't need a lot of formality or written policies. They have a clear idea of how they want things to work in their office, and they aren't the least bit shy about confronting employees who don't comply.
3. Practice owners who aren't particularly forceful or direct can achieve better cooperation from their staff by adding some formality to their management process.

Giving feedback in a constructive way

When employees don't take you seriously as a boss, it's usually because you let them know you aren't happy with their work; but, you don't do anything when it doesn't improve. Think of a parent who makes idle threats, but doesn't follow through when the kids don't eat their vegetables. And, just like your kids, you are always going to have some employees who test the boundaries of your patience

How to Measure and Improve Staff Productivity

to see how much they can get away with—it's just human nature.

So how do you give feedback in a way that establishes you as the boss, but still comes across as respectful when your employees don't meet your expectations?

The average solo practice grosses $600,000 per year and employs only four or five people. The good news is a staff that small doesn't require much formality. For that reason, I suggest that when you have a problem with someone's performance, just sit down and talk to the person. My standard phrase is to say something like this, "Mary, it's important for you to know that some things you are doing are not meeting my expectations. Let me give you some examples and tell you how I want you to handle this in the future."

I don't find it necessary to threaten, scold, or raise my voice. I just tell them in a calm way what my concern is, and I use the mirror techniques we discussed in the previous chapter to clarify they understand.

You should expect the person you are correcting to have a ready set of reasons for why they aren't performing, and I suggest that you listen politely without defending your position. It's important to stay cool and behave in an unruffled manner as though you are above the fray. That's not always easy to do, but it's your job to set the example for good

Holding Your Employees Accountable

behavior. It's important that you don't let an employee with a strong personality, or poor interpersonal skills, draw you into an argument.

If you are having employee problems and even though it might seem this way, it should not be a test of wills the same way it might be with a child or spouse. This is your practice and you don't need their permission to set certain rules. But, you do have to enforce the rules if someone is not performing the way you want them to. You're the owner or manager of this practice and if someone is not meeting your expectations in terms of job performance, you have not only a right, but an obligation, to correct them.

Also, keep in mind that addressing poor performance of any kind always extends past just one person. When someone is not pulling their weight or breaking well-established rules of the office, the other members of your staff are watching closely to see how you deal with the problem employee.

Younger ODs or those new to managing their own practice might find correcting another adult a little awkward at first, but you'll get better at it the more you do it. If this is a problem for you, just remind yourself that this person's bad attitude and weak performance is affecting not only your ability to deliver first class patient care, but also your ability to earn a living and provide for your family, not to mention the rest of your staff.

Be specific, not general with instructions

One key to being a good manager is to make sure the roles and outcomes for your office are crystal clear to everyone who works for you. Ambiguity about office policies and procedures will create a lot of confusion on the part of your staff and result in frustration for the boss and the worker. Again, doctors with a strong personality have the innate ability to be amazingly clear about the behavior they want without putting any kind of office policy in writing. Others need to add a level of formality to their process to get results.

Also, it's not fair to your staff to assume they know the 'right' way to do things in your book without clarity and feedback from you. I find it difficult to reprimand one of my team members for doing something the wrong way when I didn't fulfill my responsibility to properly inform or train them in the first place.

In his book *Switch: How To Change When Change Is Hard*, author Dan Heath advises business owners to be specific, not general, when giving instructions. He tells the story of a successful entrepreneur who owned a small remodeling business that specialized in building children's play areas. The company was known for high quality work, but, the owner was getting a lot of complaints

Holding Your Employees Accountable

from unhappy homeowners when the work crews showed up at irregular times.

In most cases, schedule changes were due to perfectly legitimate reasons such as picking up supplies, or arranging other subcontractors to meet them on the job. Unfortunately, the lack of consistent hours gave clients the impression that the workers were goofing off and could not be depended upon.

Like most optometrists, the owner of the company cared deeply how his clients felt about his service. He held meetings with the workers and told them they needed to do a better job of providing 'good customer service.' But, things didn't improve for one simple reason. His crew didn't know how to translate a general request of 'provide good customer service' into specific action steps.

Are you guilty of the same thing in your office? Do you give your employees well meaning, but general instructions like 'work hard,' 'keep busy,' or 'be nice to patients?' If you do have job descriptions, are they open ended and difficult to measure?

Back to the contractor. He wanted a tangible action that would allow his workers to better communicate their comings and goings to homeowners. So, he tried something simple.

How to Measure and Improve Staff Productivity

He instructed his crew chief to knock on the client's door each day when they arrived to inform the homeowner they were there, why they might have been delayed, and what they planned to work on that day. Customer complaints dropped immediately.

There is a lesson here for your practice—be specific, not general when giving instructions. Don't tell your staff to 'be nice' or 'work hard.' Instead, spend some time figuring out what actually constitutes 'good customer service' in your practice and give specific instructions your staff can both understand and actually do. And, strive to judge them on activities you can readily measure.

Such as, tell the receptionist at the front desk they must make eye contact and greet every patient within 60 seconds of entering the office. Another example—answer every phone call within three rings. You can also have your technician tell patients when you are running late for their exam, or call them when their glasses have been delayed more than one day at the lab.

The idea is to give instructions that translate into action steps that are easy for the staff to perform, and easy for you to measure.

The power of written feedback

At this point, let's say you do all the right things, including meeting with your problem employee to give them specific instructions on areas where their

Holding Your Employees Accountable

performance is falling short and what you want them to do about it. But, they still fall short of your expectations or, worse yet, don't take your feedback seriously. I hope this is not you, but I have seen many cases where strong willed staff members refused to do what the practice owner asked them to.

If you are one of those bosses who has trained his staff over time to know that you're all bark and no bite, your verbal feedback may not carry a lot of weight. That's the point at which you may need to start putting things in writing. There are two ways to go here—regular performance reviews, and written reprimands.

Performance reviews

Tom Peters, a well-known management consultant and best-selling author of the business classic *In Search Of Excellence*, says that the number one motivator of people is not money, but consistent and constructive feedback on their work. A great way for any practice owner to give this feedback is through written performance appraisals.

Performance appraisals give employees specific feedback on their actions and something tangible they can build on. Written reviews also provide a record of the areas discussed and provide you with a benchmark for future reviews.

How to Measure and Improve Staff Productivity

A short article in the April 2014 issue of the Management and Business Academy Newsletter stated that about 50% of all private practice optometrists did written performance appraisals with their employees, which is higher than I would have expected. While regular performance reviews are standard practice in bigger companies, the OD author described them as 'controversial' among practice owners, and said she only used performance appraisals with problem employees.

I suspect that many optometrists don't believe in doing written performance reviews on a regular basis because they view it as a punitive exercise. I have a different point of view, and I know from experience they can be a wonderful development tool if you use them on a regular basis with all your employees.

Performance reviews have been particularly helpful for me in terms of communicating difficult topics with senior team members. Yes, that can sometimes make for an uncomfortable session and it is no doubt easier to leave some issues unresolved, even if both parties are not satisfied with the situation. But, once you get things out in the open for discussion, it allows the relationship to improve and the employee to reach a new level of value to the practice. Isn't that what you want for everybody on your staff?

If you already do written performance reviews on a regular basis, I say keep it up. If you are

Holding Your Employees Accountable

considering them, I suggest you give it a try. Here are seven ways you can add a proven management tool to your practice.

1. Schedule performance reviews at twelve-month intervals for longer-term employees, and at 60 and 90 day intervals for new workers.

2. Position the review as a friendly exercise. The object of doing written performance appraisals is not to criticize, but to praise good work and, at the same time, call attention to areas that need improvement. That can be difficult to do, and impossible to document, in a conversational format.

3. If you have never done performance appraisals in your practice, one way to ease into the exercise is to have employees use your form to evaluate themselves first. You can then compare their self-appraisal with yours in a day or two. Expect some surprises!

4. Keep all of your discussions private and confidential. Performance appraisals should be done one on one, or with the office manager present.

How to Measure and Improve Staff Productivity

5. **Be sensitive to people's feelings.** Avoid writing harsh comments or exaggerating negative ratings. On the other hand, it's very important that you don't overrate mediocre employees just to be nice. An inflated good review can come back to haunt you at raise time, or if you decide to terminate a poor performer.

6. **Be realistic.** Target just two or three specific skills or areas of responsibility you want to work on, and then schedule a 30, 60, or 90 day follow-up to review improvement. For example, "Susie will learn how to do new patient work ups by December 31."

7. **Set measurable criteria for performance.** For example, 'greet all patients within 60 seconds of entering the office' or, 'complete all files by end of every work day' are far more precise than 'improve patient communications' or, 'Keep the work area clean.'

While some employers like to do performance appraisals when they do salary reviews, I recommend keeping the two processes separate. Most employees will be so focused on the size of their raise, actual performance issues may get lost in the shuffle.

Performance reviews are like advertising and marketing your practice—you won't see dramatic results the first time you do it, and it doesn't work very well if you only do it once. But, you will notice positive results if you do them on a regular basis over time.

Sample Performance Review Outline

For: _____ Date: ___ / ___ / ___

E = Exceeds Expectations
M = Meets Expectations
D = Does not meet expectations

	D	M	E
Arrives and leaves work on schedule	( )	( )	( )
Comes to work with a pleasant attitude	( )	( )	( )
Exhibits a sense of teamwork	( )	( )	( )
Dresses and groomed appropriately	( )	( )	( )
Keeps work area neat	( )	( )	( )
Quality of clerical work	( )	( )	( )
Quality of patient care	( )	( )	( )
Quality of sales skills	( )	( )	( )
Projects caring attitude to patients	( )	( )	( )
Telephone calls	( )	( )	( )
Progress on improving present skills	( )	( )	( )
and learning new skills	( )	( )	( )
Overall performance	( )	( )	( )

Comments:
_____
_____

Fig. 13

Here are some of the general areas your written

performance review should cover:

Written reprimands

I'm looking to both praise the employee and point out areas for improvement when I do a written performance review. Depending on what we have to talk about, these reviews can sometimes be uncomfortable for both me and the staff member, but I still try to position them as a friendly exercise.

Written reprimands, on the other hand, are punitive by nature as they are intended to document more egregious behavior. Example: my wife came by the office one day to see a new staff member about a small construction project the employee's boyfriend was doing for us. Their discussion escalated into an argument, and the staff member ended up shouting at my wife. She got a written reprimand and, after some discussion, we ended up letting her go.

I also had a case where a new staff member was consistently slower than expected completing her work of writing up consulting cases. This is a much more subjective situation as opposed to someone making errors in the lab. The employee's supervisor came to me to discuss the situation, and we agreed her production was below our needs for this position.

We went through the steps of documenting the issues, and gave a specific time for review. While the employee was somewhat defensive and argumentative, she did say she would make a good faith effort to work faster. Thirty days later, her production was still far below our expectations, so the supervisor and I agreed this employee was not going to work out. We gave her written notice of termination, and let her go with two weeks' notice.

When the issue is performance, it's important to document problem work habits or behavior—be specific, state exactly what the employee is doing wrong, and how that doesn't comply with your office policies. For example, let's say that Susie, the receptionist, is responsible for confirming all appointments within 24 hours of the scheduled time. But, for some reason, she isn't getting the job done and you are still having more than a normal level of no shows. Our recommendations are that you:

- Document undesirable work habit(s) or behavior
- Provide specifics steps to correct the problem
- Give a timeframe for improvement
- Schedule a follow-up meeting to review progress

If an optician continually makes clerical errors when placing jobs with the lab or ordering contact lenses, those errors result in frequent reorders that the practice pays for and will, of course, damage your reputation over time. Again, the key is written documentation—don't just make a mental note of it. Ideally, you would place a copy of the lab order in

How to Measure and Improve Staff Productivity

your file, and document the conversation you have with the employee.

Part of the reprimand process is to provide the employee with specific steps they need to take to correct the problem. For instance, if you see the error is consistently writing up jobs incorrectly for the lab, meet with them to identify the problem, and offer suggestions for improvement as well as acceptable error rates. For example, no more than one error per hundred orders over the next thirty days.

Let's look at another frequent complaint that we get from practice owners—chronic tardiness. My advice is to take the gradual approach of progressive discipline by verbally warning staff members who are chronically late. If it's just one person, you can sit down with them and say; "Diane, I have to let you know that your tardiness is a concern for me. This is just a friendly reminder, but if you don't correct the problem, I am going to put a written reprimand in your employee file."

Since it's unlikely that one warning is going to correct chronically bad behavior, you have to decide how many second chances you are going to give them before you actually write them. When the time does come, you need to call Diane in and let her know that you are documenting her tardiness and putting a written reprimand in file. The key is, don't threaten to write her up unless you intend to do it.

Holding Your Employees Accountable

Granted, this is a little harsh and in some cases is just one step shy of firing someone. But, if you're struggling to manage a certain employee you want to retain and feel they are not taking you or their job seriously, I guarantee they will pay attention the moment you put a written reprimand in their file. Formality and discipline tend to go hand in hand and the power of the pen is mighty in a case like this.

Terminating employees

About 30% of the ODs responding to a survey by the Management & Business Academy reported terminating an employee within the last twelve months. We're consultants, not attorneys so, we can't give any kind of broad legal advice on how to fire people. We do, however, have a Human Resources Consultant on staff who is available to give practice owners individual guidance in this area on a case-by-case basis.

Chapter highlights:

1. Practice owners who don't have a forceful personality can achieve better cooperation from their staff by adding some formality to their management process.
2. Regular performance evaluations are a great way for practice owners to give employee feedback in a positive and constructive way.

3. Written reprimands are punitive by nature and intended to document more egregious behavior before firing someone.

Chapter 11

Hiring Top Performers

Dear Jerry,

I seem to have a hard time hiring good people. What steps do you recommend?

Thanks,

Hiring in Hattiesburg

Hiring Top Performers

This chapter is on hiring, which means we've come full circle in our discussion about improving team productivity.

Finding good people is difficult for many private practice optometrists because we often don't start looking until we are in a bind and need somebody NOW. This, unfortunately, makes you susceptible to hiring the first decent candidate who walks through the door instead of taking the time to find a future star who can make a real difference toward building a more successful practice.

How to Stay ahead of the Recruiting Game

The reason to be proactive in your hiring process is because you KNOW you're going to be adding staff as people leave or your practice grows. For that reason, I advise you to constantly be on the lookout for good people and get in the habit of keeping a file of names with contact information when you meet impressive candidates. Excellent sources for prospects when you're not actually looking to hire somebody are:

1. Existing patients. Some doctors are shy about doing this, but this was a great source for me and I always made a point to hire people who wore glasses and contacts. Whenever I found

How to Measure and Improve Staff Productivity

myself in the exam room with a sharp person who was currently working in a job that paid similar to my office, I would put their name on my list of future prospects.
2. Retail clerks who you meet in a store, and sales people who call on you. The best office manager I ever had called on me as a rep for an office supply company before I hired him away.
3. Sharp waiters and waitresses who may be moonlighting, and looking for a better day job.

If you're impressed with someone who waits on you in a store or restaurant, you might ask innocently what their name is and how long they've worked there. You can give your card, or make a note to yourself for future reference.

Of course, the standard option when you need to hire somebody is to advertise in the help wanted section of the local newspaper, or online sources like Craigslist. I've had surprisingly good luck there also. The headline and wording of your ad is critically important to generate good responses. Doctor's Office is much better than something like Help Wanted for example. I make a point to use key phrases such as 'pleasant work environment,' opportunity for advancement,' and 'attractive compensation and benefits.'

Not everybody agrees, but I like to include an hourly rate in my ads. You have to be competitive for your community if you want to hire good people and that information will attract the applicants in your price range. This also allows candidates with higher salary demands to eliminate themselves on the front end.

I run so called 'blind ads' which means my name is not mentioned for confidentiality reasons, and I really don't want to get inundated with calls by unqualified job seekers. Many doctors openly ask friends and colleagues for referrals, but I prefer to be discreet and I avoid this approach because it can be awkward when friends and patients (whom you have no interest in hiring) call you looking for a job.

How to Screen a Group of Résumés

In most cases, résumés will come in by email, and you'll get thirty or forty if you're lucky. If you've written an appealing ad, you can count on about 80% of your applicants being not even close to what you are looking for. When I am reviewing résumés and personal history, I print out the ones of interest and look at educational background and special academic honors, job tenure in previous positions, quality of previous positions, and proximity to my office. I try to identify applicants who've done well in high school or college, and I don't want to hire someone who may find the commute onerous after the newness of the job wears off. Salary requirements are important, and we've already covered how to determine if someone's personal income requirements fit your practice budget in Chapter 5.

Once I start evaluating a stack of résumés, I try to rank them as objectively as possible and assign each one a grade such as:

A = must talk to

B = maybe

C = not for me

I'll hand write that grade at the top of the first page of the résumé so I don't waste time reviewing ones I've already ruled out. To be sure, it's an imperfect system and judgment always plays an important role—the good news is you get better at it the more you do.

After I rank my résumés, I'll pick my five or six best candidates, and personally call them to set up phone interviews. I'll introduce myself by saying something such as, "Hi, Ms. Smith, this is Dr. Hayes. I'm calling in reference to the résumé you sent for the position in the doctor's office I advertised on Craigslist. Is this a good time to talk, or should we set up another call?"

I prefer to do a phone interview before seeing them in person for a couple of reasons: I can spend less time with someone who doesn't impress me, and

Hiring Top Performers

I am more objective on the phone than when I am sitting with someone face to face. I find the process is more effective if I start out by asking everyone the

---

Job Interview Notes

Candidate Name: _____ Date: / /

Tell me about your work experience.
_____
_____

Do you wear glasses or contact lenses?
_____

What strengths do you bring to the work place?
_____
_____

How would your boss and co-workers describe you?
_____
_____

Describe a project or job you did really well.
_____
_____

What areas do you think you need to improve in?
_____
_____

What appeals to you about this position?
_____
_____

Comments and impressions:
_____

---

same questions, so I make up a little form to give the interview some structure.

Fig. 14

How to Measure and Improve Staff Productivity

Once I've talked to my best prospects on the phone, I create a matrix with a horizontal list of candidates by name, and a vertical list of the criteria I am looking for such as the sample below. I then use this as a way to compare my top candidates on paper.

Job Candidate Matrix

	Candidate 1	Candidate 2	Candidate 3	Candidate 4	Candidate 5
Name	Mary	Kayla	Thomas	Susie	Heather
General work experience					
Optical experience					
Sales experience					
Healthcare Experience					
Phone voice					
Wears glasses or contacts					
Drive time from the office					
Their interest in the job					
Salary expectations					
Intangibles					
Overall general impression					
My interest in hiring them					
Comments:					

Fig. 15

How to do personal interviews

At this point, I have narrowed the field to my two (three, if I'm lucky) top prospects, and I am ready to set up personal interviews in the office. I like to spend time with the candidate one on one before I have them get the once over from the rest of my staff. I'll start with open-ended questions such as, "Where are you from originally?" and "How long have you lived in this area?" That helps them get settled and comfortable. Then I'll review key questions from the phone interview about their skill set and work history.

I think it's important to ask tough questions to see how a prospect handles themselves under fire. Google reportedly quizzes young tech geniuses during job interviews by asking crazy questions such how many gas stations there are in the United States. They don't expect someone to know trivia like that, they just want to see their thought process.

You can do your own version of this exercise by asking your candidates open-ended questions about how they would handle hypothetical service issues. For example:

- What would you do if a patient were complaining that they couldn't see out of

their new glasses in front of everyone in the reception area?
- What would you do if someone told you they didn't have their insurance card with them, but they needed to seen today?

You don't expect them to know the right answers for your office—you just want to see their thought processes. The point is, the purpose of the in-office personal interview is more for the candidate to convince me they are worth hiring than for me to sell them on the idea of coming to work for me.

Perhaps the most common mistake I see during the personal interview process is employers who are so proud of what they do, and they go overboard with the show and tell mode. I've been guilty of this myself many times. I've also seen enthusiastic managers who worked for me talk at a candidate for fifteen minutes non-stop, and go into a level of detail about the job no one could possibly grasp in one sitting. Remember, this is an interview, not a training session, and you won't learn much about the candidate if you do most of the talking.

My strong advice is to develop the mindset that you want the candidate to do at least 60% of the talking. Otherwise, they are going to leave your office impressed with you, but you'll be scratching your head trying to remember what you liked about them.

Hiring Top Performers

The importance of pre-hire testing

I went through a string of bad hires early in my career which lead to the realization that candidates who present themselves with a well-written résumé and good references often interview better than they perform in the job once you actually hire them. It's called the 'Halo Effect.' An attractive, well spoken, enthusiastic candidate can make a great first impression, even when their skills do not fit your needs.

A great way to add some objectivity beyond your own intuition to your interview process is to require all candidates to take some sort of standardized test. I started with the Wonderlic Personnel Test years ago which is a great tool to gauge someone's basic aptitude (www.wonderlic.com). Typical questions might be something like, "How long would it take to drive 100 miles if you are going 30 MPH?" The test comes with a scale telling you what range a person should score in depending the position they are interviewing for. That might be 20 for a receptionist, and 35 for an engineer.

I also like to use some type of personality assessment tool to find out if the person we are considering hiring is more of a introvert, extrovert, or somewhere in between. You want to know that because an introverted person will do fine as a billing

How to Measure and Improve Staff Productivity

clerk or bookkeeper, but their natural position would not be as a front desk receptionist answering the phone, and dealing with patients all day. Likewise, a caring and efficient chairside scribe may lack the natural aptitude for sales that you want the frame stylist in your optical dispensary to have. Prima offers a variety of assessments you can use with both new hires and existing employees.

Hire slow, fire fast as some consultants like to say.

Experience versus talent

There is an ongoing debate as to whether it's better to hire someone of average skills who brings experience to the job, or an obviously sharp applicant with an outgoing personality who is bright and eager to learn? I like to surround myself with the best people I can find—so, I believe in the old saying *hire for personality and aptitude, and train for specific skills.* You want a pleasant, outgoing person at your front desk, regardless of his or her past optical experience. The same holds true for all the positions that work directly with patients such as technicians and scribes. You can teach the skills you need for most positions, but you're not going to train a negative person with a sour personality to be pleasant and outgoing in your office no matter how smart they are.

The level of experience you need in a candidate also depends on how technical the position, and how long it might take someone to learn it. For positions that require formal training or licensure such as a bench optician or billing and coding clerk, I would attempt to hire based on past experience and current competence. It also depends greatly on what you are good at. Every OD can teach a sharp novice how to do case histories, pretests, and scribing. Likewise, a doctor who knows how to run an optical lab might be perfectly comfortable training a new hire to cut and edge.

Hiring on a trial basis

Depending on the laws in your state, it can be a good idea to bring new hires in on a 60 - 90 day probationary basis. You can set a mandatory date to do a performance review, and make a decision on them at that point.

Zappos™, the wildly successful online shoe and clothing company owned by Amazon™, has an interesting policy—they put all new hires through a four week program on policies, procedures, and culture. When that training period is over, new employees get what is known as 'the offer'—if you quit today, we will pay you for the time worked, PLUS a bonus of $5,000!

They started the program with $1,000 and it worked so well, they gradually increased the amount.

That's strong! But, it really helps weed out the people who are there just for the paycheck.

Chapter highlights:

1. Stay on the lookout for good people, and get in the habit of keeping a file of names with contact information when you meet impressive candidates.
2. The hiring process generally consists of five steps: finding good candidates, screening résumés, phone interviews, personal interviews, and then the offer.
3. I believe in the old saying, *hire for personality and aptitude, and train for specific skills.*

Epilogue

Success Secrets of High Producing ODs

Dear Jerry,

I know there is a lot that goes into having a successful private practice. In your experience, what are the two or three things that really separate the high producers from the average practice?

Ambitious in Atlanta

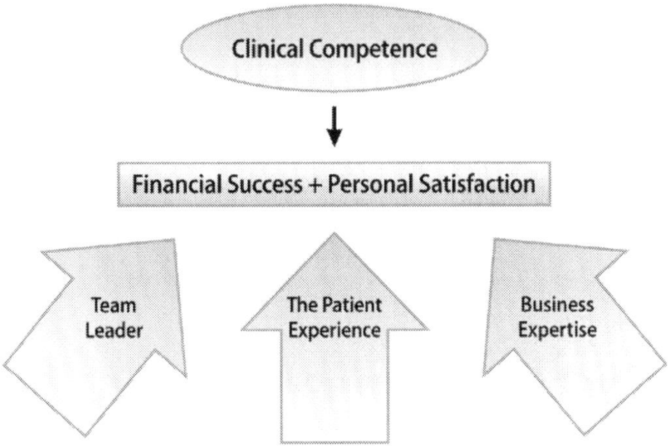

Epilogue

```
        ┌─────────────────────┐
        │  Clinical Competence │
        └─────────────────────┘
                   ↓
    ┌──────────────────────────────────────┐
    │ Financial Success + Personal Satisfaction │
    └──────────────────────────────────────┘

    ⬆ Team        ⬆ The Patient      ⬆ Business
      Leader        Experience         Expertise
```

Four keys to success in private practice

Fig. 16

As I mentioned earlier, there are four key areas that you must master at some level if you want to be successful in private practice. Clinical competence is not enough.

When an otherwise good doctor is struggling to grow revenues and he is not feeling very satisfied as a practice owner, it's often because he overemphasizes the clinical side of the practice. I recognize that may sound counterintuitive—but, if you're not paying enough attention to team leadership and providing a positive experience for your patients, as well as

How to Measure and Improve Staff Productivity

staying on top of the financial side of practice, you won't be as busy or profitable as your more business savvy colleagues. We'll have more to say on those topics in the upcoming book that Nathan Hayes, Prima's Practice Finance Consultant, and I are writing now—*Success Secrets of High Producing ODs.*

JERRY HAYES, OD
Prima Eye Group, LLC
jerryhayesod.com
jhayes@primaeyegroup.com

CHRYSALIS PUBLISHING AUTHOR SERVICES
Editor: L.A. O'Neil
chrysalispub@gmail.com

GRAPHICS
John Roquet

Made in the USA
Lexington, KY
14 September 2014